For Bill Lewis—fitness guru and tremendously
special friend. Thank you.

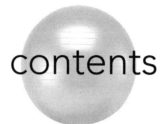

contents

Acknowledgments   vii

Introduction   ix
Why I love fitness balls, and why you'll love them, too!

PART ONE: THE WORKOUT

Chapter 1: A Well-Rounded Start   3
Everything you need to start your journey to a beautiful body

Chapter 2: Best Ball Exercises for a Beautiful Body   27
Target your arms, abs, back, shoulders, thighs, and butt in less than 30 minutes a session

Chapter 3: Building Your Confidence   71
Challenging tips, tricks, and exercises to push your fitness to the next level

PART TWO: THE SIX-WEEK BODY MAKEOVER

Chapter 4: Your Six-Week Body Makeover   93
The elements of success

Chapter 5: Why Every Dieter Needs Dessert   101
And why reduced fat and nonfat foods just don't cut the mustard

Chapter 6: Working Up a Sweat   **129**
*Pairing your ball workout with aerobic exercise helps you achieve
faster results*

Chapter 7: Your Six-Week Workbook   **137**
*Day-by-day tips, workouts, and eating goals to help
you stay on track*

PART THREE: YOUR PERSONAL APPROACH

Chapter 8: Six Weeks and Beyond   245
*Customizing your ball routine to your personal interests
and needs to help you stick with the program for life*

Chapter 9: A Ball for Every Body   253
*Play tennis? Need an exercise partner? Short on time?
Find a customized ball routine that's exactly right for you!*

PART FOUR: BEAUTIFUL FOR LIFE

Chapter 10: When Life Intervenes   275
*How to follow your ball program and dessert diet at restaurants,
at work, when traveling, and when under stress*

Chapter 11: Motivated For Life   285
*Spice up your program with plenty of variety, and you'll
never fall off the ball*

Chapter 12: Partner Pointers   291
*Your social network greatly influences whether you'll
stick with your new habits*

Chapter 13: Beautiful Body, Beautiful Mind   297
*Maximize your brainpower, and you'll also maximize your
motivation, happiness, and inner beauty*

Index   307

About the Author   315

Bounce
Your Body
Beautiful

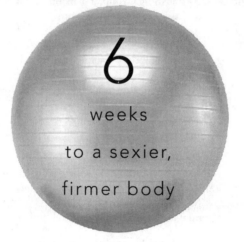

6

weeks

to a sexier,

firmer body

LIZ APPLEGATE, PH.D.

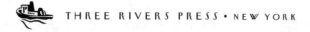

THREE RIVERS PRESS • NEW YORK

Published by Three Rivers Press, New York, New York.
Member of the Crown Publishing Group, a division of Random House, Inc.
www.randomhouse.com

THREE RIVERS PRESS and the Tugboat design are
registered trademarks of Random House, Inc.

Originally published by Prima Publishing, Roseville, California, in 2003.

Design by Melanie Haage Design

Illustrations by Michael Tanamachi

Photographs by Liz Reap
All photographs courtesy of Ball Dynamics International, Inc.
(800-752-2255, www.balldynamics.com)

Printed in the United States of America

Library of Congress Cataloging-in-Publication Data
Applegate, Elizabeth Ann.
Bounce your body beautiful : six weeks to a sexier, firmer body /
Liz Applegate.— 1st ed.
p.   cm.
Includes index.
1. Exercise for women. 2. Balls (Sporting goods) 3. Physical fitness for women.
I. Title.
GV482 .A66   2002

613.7'045—dc21   2002151818

ISBN 0-7615-1563-1
10 9 8 7 6 5 4 3

First Edition

acknowledgments

While sitting back (on my fitness ball, of course) and reviewing this book before it goes off to press, I reflect on the generous support and expert efforts that so many people provided in bringing this book to fruition. Thanks first go to Bill Lewis, my medical rehabilitation exercise specialist, who got me back on my feet after many surgeries and injuries and, as a result, introduced me to the powers of fitness balls. Thank you, Bill, for your expert rehab training, warm encouragement, and great friendship. My huge thanks go to Alisa Bauman whose tremendous writing, organizational, and creative efforts made this book a reality. You're the best, Alisa. Thank you to Marlia Braun, whose advice and expertise on the nutritional analysis was so valuable.

During this project, I learned that vivid and concise photos are a must. And in a fitness book such as this a great deal of work goes into the planning and execution of the photographs. The photography in this book is excellent, and I thank Liz Reap for such a superb job. Her keen eye, fast finger-clicking, and patience made for truly great photos. And so many thanks go to her assistant Ryan Hulvat for his help and expertise and to his assistant Gary who painstakingly kept the wrinkles out of my outfits during each photo. Jennifer McKeever, who did the make-up and styling, did a fabulous job. I also thank Nike's Women's Technical Training and Studio line as well as Sugoi for wonderful clothing and shoes worn in the photos. And many thanks to Ball Dynamics International, Inc., for their generous support of the photo shoot and for supplying the heavy balls and fitness balls throughout the development of my program and book.

My warm thanks also go to the many friends and fitness-minded folks who tried out my Bounce Your Body Beautiful program and provided me with great feedback: Kris Clark, Karen Schelegle, Karen Galbreath, Susan Munn, and Stu Kahn—the head coach for Davis Aquadart Swim team—among many others.

So many more people assisted me with this tremendous effort, including my literary agent Laurie Harper, who had great vision and passion about my program. My assistants Jessica Callaghan and Jennifer Bergfeld did nothing short of miraculous work in helping me meet deadlines. They also graciously dealt with every crisis (of which there were a few!)—thanks so much to the two of you. Prior to the book's release, a Web site (www.lizapplegate.com) was set up by the talented designer Glenn Hughes. Thanks Glenn for bringing so much excitement to this book. Thanks also go to my editors at Prima, Denise Sternad and Tara Joffe, who not only pulled this book together but also share my enthusiasm about the benefits of fitness balls. And thank you Grant, Natalie, Mark, Millie, and Rocko for your support and caring.

introduction

Why I love fitness balls, and why you'll love them, too!

I bought my first fitness ball during the 1980s when my son, Grant, experienced difficulty learning to walk. Our family doctor and physical therapist recommended exercises with a large, vinyl, air-filled ball to help Grant improve his balance and muscle coordination.

At the time, fitness balls were used exclusively to help children improve their neurological skills. I began with Grant by draping his tiny body over the ball and using one hand on his back to steady him and the other to move the ball from side to side. Grant loved it and smiled and giggled as he did his "workout." He soon advanced to standing on the ball as I twisted it from side to side.

Then, one day, at 20 months, Grant walked.

I kept that large green ball in our living room for a few years as a symbol of Grant's achievement until at age 5 Grant challenged the ball to a sword fight. As you can imagine, the old ball didn't stand a chance. Just one jab with Grant's play sword, and that ball was history.

I didn't give the use of fitness balls another thought until about twelve years later when I was recuperating from shoulder surgery. By that time, exercises incorporating fitness balls had become the standard rehabilitation treatment for almost every injury, from shoulder pain to back woes. They were also coming into use for physical fitness. They had come out of the closet and were in just about every gym, promoted as the latest way to sculpt rock-hard abs.

Called everything from the Swiss ball to the stability ball to the balance ball to the gymnastic ball to the fit ball, fitness balls had become mainstream. They can now be found all over, in gyms, stores, and homes.

My physical therapist told me that my exercises with the fitness ball would not only help me retrain the muscles in my injured shoulder but would also help me get in the best shape of my life. I was skeptical. Before my shoulder injury, I had stayed fit with a hardcore program of chin-ups, push-ups, bench presses, and other traditional gym exercises. I also swam, ran, and cycled almost every day. With this complete regimen, I doubted that exercises using a fitness ball and light resistance could do as much or more for me.

I have a doctorate in nutrition with a specialization in exercise physiology, I teach nutrition at the University of California, Davis, and I consult with NBA and NFL teams. I decided to treat the ball as a fitness experiment—one that I assumed would serve as entertaining fodder when teaching or counseling athletes. I never imagined that I'd soon find myself suggesting the fitness ball program to all, including students, athletes, and friends.

By the end of my shoulder rehab program, I was fitter and more svelte than I'd been in my life. That's saying a lot, given I competed as a professional triathlete during my twenties and early thirties.

Every time I looked in the mirror, I was amazed at how toned I had become, even though I am in my forties. Over time, I slowly eased my way back into the swimming pool and realized how my improved balance and coordination were helping me swim with a more efficient stroke and do more powerful flip turns. Not only did I swim like a pro, but I also looked and felt fantastic.

I never went back to my old fitness equipment. My son inherited my set of dumbbells, and I began hanging wet towels on my free-standing chin-up bar as I walked through my garage. One day, I'll donate my barbell weight plates to charity, but for now I use them to hold my fitness ball in place when I'm not using it.

Meanwhile, friends were noticing my improved physique as well as my great attitude. When I credited the fitness ball with my renewed strength, toned muscles, and energy, they couldn't believe it. They had seen these balls at their gyms and at stores, but they didn't know their purpose or what to do with them. So I invited a few friends over and showed them some exercises.

Like me, in the beginning they were skeptical. "This ball is just good for working your abs, right?" Jennifer asked me.

"No, you'll use it to tone and firm your entire body," I replied.

"You must still do more than only work on the ball. You also use dumbbells, right?" Linda asked.

"Nope. Just the big fitness ball and these handheld heavy balls."

I showed them a series of exercises. By the end of the workout, my friends told me that, for the first time in their lives, they felt they had truly worked every muscle in their bodies.

In just a few weeks they noticed other changes. Their bodies were more firm, and they felt more balanced. Word got out. My good friend Kris in Pennsylvania begged me to show her some moves. Even the local youth and masters swim teams wanted to get on the ball. Delighted, I showed them some routines, and the swimmers have been on the ball ever since.

"Most of the girls, even those with superior swimming skills, had coordination difficulties when they first began our exercise program," says Stu, head swim coach for the Davis Aquadart Age Group Swim Team. "However, as the girls became more accomplished on the fitness balls, I saw a corresponding increase in their skills in the pool. They actually began to swim differently, with more control."

Without exception, everyone who tried the ball program raved about it.

One of these enthusiasts was my good friend Karen, a pediatric nurse and mother of three teens, who marveled at the increase in balance, muscle tone, and core body strength she experienced after starting her fitness ball routine.

"It really strengthened the core of my body, up and down my spine, and markedly improved my flexibility," she says. "The ball work has improved my posture, diminished my nagging and draining lower back and shoulder and neck pains, improved my stamina, and given me a much more positive and confident physical presence. I love doing the ball exercises. They give me a sense of inner physical power!"

The Amazing Ball Workout

Why does the fitness ball provide such amazing results for so many women? Let me count the ways.

1. **Fitness balls provide a more efficient workout compared to weight machines and dumbbells.** In fact, a recent study from the University of Waterloo in Ontario, Canada, found that people who did curl-up abdominal exercises on a ball rather than on the floor doubled the tension on their rectus abdominus—the large muscle that forms your "six pack"—and quadrupled the activity of their obliques—the muscles that form the sides of your abdomen and waist.

The secret? The inherent instability of the ball's round surface. When you work out with dumbbells and a bench or with exercise machines, you primarily use only the muscle you are focusing on. When you do a biceps curl, you only work your biceps. But when you do that same move on a fitness ball, you must use the muscles in your legs, abdomen, buttocks, and back just to stay balanced. These muscles keep you from falling off the ball. With no other exercise equipment do you work so many muscles at once.

As recent ball convert Julie in Pennsylvania put it, "No other exercise has ever worked my butt while I'm targeting my chest or upper body."

2. **Fitness balls encourage you to be consistent.** Because you can keep your fitness ball at home, deflate it and pack it in a suit-

case, and generally use it anywhere you find yourself, you'll never have an excuse to skip a workout.

"I'll be taking my exercise ball with me on vacation this summer, since it's so simple to transport and the exercises are so easy to re-member and fun to do," said my good friend Karen, a veterinary inten-sive case unit nurse. "It's portable, economical, user-friendly, versatile, fun, and fabulous. I love it!"

We've all seen how often people set up their home gyms in a dreary basement or garage, not because these dark, lonely places inspire fit-ness, but because a weight bench and dumbbells take up a lot of room and don't really go with the living room décor. Not so your fitness ball. It fits in just fine anywhere, allowing you to do your workout in the liv-ing room or even in the backyard. On a beautiful day, you can roll the ball outside and do your moves as you breathe in the fresh air.

My friend Alisa does her fitness ball exercises while she watches *Oprah*. "I get a better workout than I otherwise would at the gym," she tells me. "At the gym I'm always thinking, 'How fast can I get this over with?' But when I'm at home, I tend to add extra exercises or do more sets or reps in order to drag out my session to match the full hour of the *Oprah* show."

3. Everyone benefits from using fitness balls. There are no cumbersome weights to maneuver. Anyone—from an 80-year-old woman to a young child—can exercise with a fitness ball. And, instead of hoisting heavy barbells and dumbbells for resistance, you work with small "heavy balls" that everyone can lift. These "heavy balls" are handheld, water-filled balls that offer lighter resistance than other weights, thus making your workout safer. These smaller balls also increase your grip strength. They allow you to put your muscles through a greater range of motion, and they encourage you to complete more repetitions at a lower weight, a big factor in sculpting the long, lean muscle look that many women seek.

4. Balls make working out feel fun and natural. Fitness balls and the handheld balls bring back fond childhood memories, whereas dumbbells tend to make women feel unfeminine and tense. Just about every kid in American has bounced or thrown a ball, whereas few women grew up with a set of dumbbells.

As one of my clients, Lori, put it, "It's a blast. I just feel good balancing on the ball."

Why Strength for Women?

You now know why fitness balls provide the best tool for strengthening and toning your muscles, but if working out is all new to you, you may be wondering why you need to strengthen your muscles at all when your primary goal is really weight loss.

For years women focused on cardiovascular exercise mostly in the form of aerobics classes as their primary weight-loss tool. Only recently have they become aware that, to truly firm up and lose weight, they must also strength train.

Research shows that our sedentary lives cause us to lose 1 to 2 pounds of muscle during each decade of life after age 20. Each pound of muscle we have left burns roughly 35 to 50 calories a day doing "muscle maintenance" that involves breaking itself down and building itself back up. This means that every pound of muscle we lose slows our metabolism by 35 to 50 calories a day.

You might not notice this metabolism slowdown in your twenties or even in your thirties, but by your forties or fifties, you may be burning 200 to 300 fewer calories a day than you did in your twenties. That's one less Snickers bar or McDonald's milkshake you can eat or drink in a day. Because most of us fail to adjust our diets and eat less food as our metabolism slows, we see the results in wider thighs and thicker waistlines. We bemoan the fact that this extra weight becomes harder and harder to take off.

Yet you can reverse this metabolism slowdown. The answer? You guessed it—strength training.

When a muscle meets resistance, its fibers first break down and then build back up. When the fibers build back up, they grow in size and strength to face that same task without strain. This larger size bolsters muscle strength as well as your metabolism, which is the number of calories that your body burns just to exist.

Muscles burn a number of calories simply to maintain themselves. The larger your muscle fibers, the more calories the muscle will burn. A typical woman starting a strength program can add 1 to 2 pounds of muscle, creating a permanent metabolism boost of 35 to 75 calories or more per day.

To see how powerful this metabolism boost is, here's a story about my friend Kris and me. We were walking through the exhibitor's area at an international sports medicine conference one morning and stopped to watch one of the exhibitors demonstrating a new device that measured resting metabolic rate.

Both Kris and I decided to give it a try. Kris sat in the chair, put the mask over her face, and a few minutes later learned that she burned 1470 calories a day just by breathing, digesting, and living. That was a fantastic 14 percent above the norm for her age.

I sat in the chair, put the mask over my face, and soon learned that my *resting* rate was 2100 calories, 70 percent above the norm. That was even more amazing!

Both Kris and I exercise regularly except that I strength train a bit more consistently than she does. My strength training proved its worth in my metabolic rate.

Kris and I, in our forties, both are living proof that metabolism doesn't have to slow with age, providing you feed it with the right kind of exercise to keep it running.

Besides boosting metabolism, larger muscle fibers give shape to our abs, buns, and arms, all without making us look bulky.

Some women worry that performing a resistance exercise means they'll develop masculine-looking muscles. I'll let you in on a secret.

Many of those women that you see in muscle magazines didn't get that way naturally. They used steroids, the male hormone testosterone, to get their muscles to grow that large.

The vast majority of women don't have the genetics or the hormonal profile to develop that size muscle. Even if you are one of the few women with the genetic tendency to grow large muscles, you don't have to worry. The specific nature of the ball program prevents large muscle growth. With its focus on numerous repetitions rather than heavy weights, the ball program always sculpts sleek, beautiful, feminine muscles.

In addition to building larger muscle fibers, a resistance program also increases the protein content of your muscles so that your connective tissue—tendons, cartilage, and ligaments—becomes thicker and stronger. This means that in addition to having more strength, you will also be preventing injuries.

More muscle strength also gives you more coordination. Finally, resistance training also helps bones preserve their mineral content, a factor in preventing fractures as we age.

Possibly most important of all, having strength is empowering. You'll soon be able to do things that you thought you needed to ask men to do. You'll open tight jars, lift heavy water jugs, carry groceries without a cart, and more. Within your own fitness routine, you'll feel inspired each time you add more push-ups or more reps or weight to a particular exercise.

Being strong feels good. You feel capable. You begin to move with confidence and ease. Best of all, you look fabulous.

Making the Most of the Program

Throughout this book, I provide you with numerous routines. After you read chapter 1 and find out what you need to get started, I suggest you begin in one of two places.

The Basic Program   Chapter 2 describes the basic ball routines and covers a span of six weeks. If you've never lifted weights before, start here. These exercises will help you build strength, coordination, and balance. You'll notice that the routines change every two weeks. Switching your exercises will help keep your muscles constantly challenged and will also increase your calorie burn during your workouts.

The Body Makeover   My body makeover in part 2 takes the basic exercises introduced in chapter 2 and combines them with a nutrition guide and cardiovascular exercises that are designed to help you lose weight and completely make over your body. If you are motivated to make several changes at once—both in your diet and your fitness routine—this is a great place to start. It's also a great program if you are the type of person who needs to follow a blueprint to help you exercise and eat right. The body makeover gives you a 42-day exercise and eating program and holds your hand every step of the way.

Both programs last six weeks, the amount of time most people need to see noticeable results. By the end of the program you choose, you will feel stronger and look slimmer and more toned. You'll also radiate new confidence.

Because of the efficient nature of the ball workout, my routines take fewer than 30 minutes. Most women tell me they are able to fit in the workout in the morning before work, during a lunch break, or in between cooking tasks before dinner.

That said, I have to warn you that your first workout will probably take more than 30 minutes, because you will need extra time to read the exercise descriptions and to experiment with different body positions. If you are short on time, try doing half the exercises one day and the other half the next day. As you gain proficiency with the movements, you'll soon find that you can do the entire workout in less than 30 minutes.

Once you have completed either the basic ball program or the six-week body makeover, you can move on to either chapter 3 or 9.

- Chapter 3 will increase the difficulty of your ball workout. Simply put, the more challenging your workout, the better your results. Challenging yourself with tougher ball moves will keep your workouts mentally entertaining as well as fuel your confidence. Many of these exercises build on moves you learn in chapter 2. I recommend you start with chapter 2 and master those moves before moving on to the routine in chapter 3.

- Chapter 9 provides specific ball exercises for various goals and lifestyles. If you're looking for ways to improve your tennis or golf game, you'll find them here. If you want some help targeting your body's trouble spots, head to this chapter. If you need ideas on how to do the ball program with your family or children, turn here. You can incorporate these exercises into the routine you learn in chapter 2.

In addition to ball exercises and eating plans, this book offers a wealth of motivational tips to take you beyond the six-week programs and help you stick with the ball program for life. You'll learn how to customize your program to your personal needs and time constraints, how to stick to your program when traveling and when under stress, how to gain more support from those around you, and how to use your mind to better fuel your motivation.

What to Expect Week by Week

As soon as you start your ball program, you will feel your body transform, even during your very first workout.

Whenever you make your body stretch in order to accomplish something—for example, lifting a heavy weight—it undergoes some changes that make your next attempt that much easier. During your first workout, you will feel awkward. That's great. That means your muscles are working *hard* to keep you balanced. It also means your muscles are recruiting large amounts of their fiber to do the exercise and are causing you to burn calories.

By the end of week 1, you should feel more confident and balanced on the ball. You'll also feel exhilarated. You will have mastered many different movements. You'll be amazed at your body's ability to learn and your ability to stick to a fun new program.

By the end of week 2, you'll notice a definite increase in strength. You'll find that you can increase the number of repetitions in all of the exercises. During week 3, you'll learn an entirely new set of exercises and will again experience the exhilaration that comes from discovering the natural wisdom of your body.

By week 4 you'll have gained enough strength to cut back on your rest break between exercises and sets and thus speed up your workout. You'll feel less fatigue during your ball workout and in going about the activities of daily life. You'll also feel more balanced and coordinated.

By weeks 5 and 6 you'll begin to feel like a new woman in a new body. You'll see muscle definition. You'll notice slimmer thighs and a slimmer waistline. Your increased strength will allow you to accomplish more tasks during the day. You'll find you can open stubborn jar tops. You'll climb stairs without feeling winded. You'll carry grocery bags and not notice the weight. You'll lift your kids to your shoulder and not complain about their ever-growing bodies!

I hope you will be as excited as I am about *Bounce Your Body Beautiful*. Let's get started!

PART ONE

the workout

1

a well-rounded start

Everything you need to start your journey to a beautiful body

I'm so excited to bring you the Bounce Your Body Beautiful program, the most effective toning workout for women. In just six weeks you'll tone sleek muscles, improve your balance and coordination, strengthen your abdomen, feel stronger, increase your coordination, and look radiant.

The ball workout provides an amazing, fun, and convenient exercise method. Best of all, it's designed to work on a woman's unique body proportions and to fit in with her lifestyle.

As I mentioned in the introduction, I discovered the amazing nature of these large, vinyl, air-filled balls when I was recuperating from shoulder surgery. At the time, I could not continue my standard routine, which included chin-ups, bench presses, and other hard-core moves, because it would have damaged my shoulder.

Bill, my certified medical rehab trainer, recommended a routine on the fitness ball, and I've been on it ever since! The workout has transformed my body. It will do the same for you!

One great aspect of the ball program is that it's so easy to get started. Unlike other programs, it doesn't require a cumbersome and expensive home gym. My ball workout has just three pieces of equipment: the fitness ball, some heavy balls, and an exercise mat. Here's what to look for in each.

The Fitness Ball   You can find fitness balls just about everywhere these days, including sporting goods stores. You can also shop online at www.balldynamics.com. Though you'll find numerous brands, I prefer the Gymnic fitness balls. I find them to be more durable and more comfortable than other types. Other brands include Fitball, Duraball, and Gymnastic, among others. The balls range in cost from about $20 to about $50.

Fitness balls come in a variety of sizes. The right ball for you allows you to sit down with your knees bent at 90-degree angles. In general, the ball sizes work for the heights as shown in figure 1.1.

The Heavy Balls   You will need weighted balls for some, but not all, of the exercises in my program. The heavy balls, which are filled with water, add resistance to particular exercises that target your upper arms and shoulders. You can use dumbbells or even large soup cans if you prefer. However, the heavy balls make your workout more effective. Simply grabbing them increases your grip strength, which is so useful in opening stubborn jar tops. Also, curling and pressing a ball recruits numerous smaller muscles to help stabilize your hands, thus increasing the efficiency of your workout. Finally, the round shape of the heavy

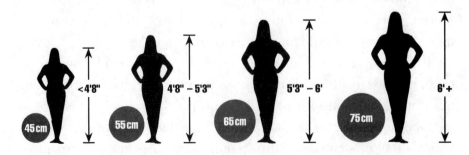

Figure 1.1

balls fits perfectly into a woman's smaller hands and feels more natural than dumbbells, with their cold feel, metallic smell, and callus-inflicting roughness.

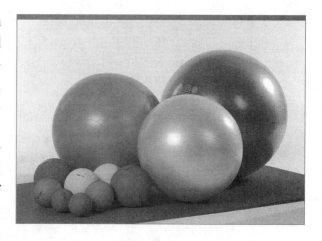

When choosing heavy balls, take your fitness level and hand size into account. If you decide to go with Gymnic heavy balls, note that the green ball is the size of a softball and weighs 1.1 pounds. Most women can lift this weight, and it fits their palm and gives a good grip. The balls increase in size by an inch and are color-coded from red to yellow to blue to orange. Most women do just fine with green, yellow, or red.

The Mat   Your mat serves two purposes. First, it holds your feet and hands in place, preventing them from sliding out from under you during certain exercises. Second, it acts as a cushion, allowing you to lie or kneel comfortably on the floor. Look for a mat that fits your body size. For example, I'm just over 5 feet tall, so I use a mat that's 2 feet by 6 feet. If you're much taller or have extra weight to lose, you might need a mat that's a little wider or longer, but you won't need one any larger than 3 feet by 7 feet.

Look for a mat with a nubby surface designed to reduce slippage. If you buy your mat at a sporting goods store, test it by pressing your hands into it. If your hands slide, the mat isn't sticky enough.

Getting Acquainted with the Ball

Once you have your equipment, you're ready to roll—literally.

When you first work out on the ball, you *will* feel awkward. Rest assured that this is normal. Your body is simply learning a new way to

Just Sit on It

The more you use the ball, the more likely you'll stick to your new routine.

Fortunately, the ball has numerous uses.

For one, the ball works as a great chair. Sit on it whenever you can. Use it as a prop when watching TV. Sit on it and let your company use the couch or easy chair! Use it as a desk chair. Sitting on the ball will provide a mini workout as you use your abdominal muscles to remain upright. Plus, you won't be able to resist the urge to wiggle and move, which will help burn a few extra calories.

You can also use the ball as a toy and fitness tool for small children. Roll it back and forth to your toddler. Place your toddler on top, put one hand on your toddler's back and the other on the ball, and move the ball as your toddler works on balance.

The ball also makes a wonderful footrest. Keep it in plain view. Use it and you won't lose it!

move. Eventually, your brain and muscles will adapt to the new movement, and your sessions will feel more natural.

You can cut down on some of that awkwardness and increase your inner confidence by treating your first workout as a "get acquainted" session.

To start, put on some fun music and place the ball near a wall. Sit on the ball, with your back to the wall. Wiggle around, moving your buttocks from left to right and your torso from side to side, all while keeping to the beat of the music. Bounce up and down. Spend a minute or two getting used to the sensation of sitting on the ball.

Next, try balancing. Lift one foot off the floor. Once you get the hang of it, try lifting both feet. Don't worry about falling. You can always lean into the wall behind you or lower your feet. This little exercise helps eliminate any fear of falling off the ball and builds your confidence. It also gives you a great core workout.

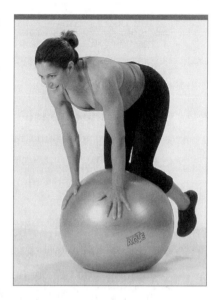

On your first try you may wonder if you'll ever get the hang of it. Trust me, you will. Feel the ball wobble. Feel your abdomen work to pull the ball back into position.

Once you feel comfortable sitting on the ball, try a slightly harder balancing exercise. Kneel with your palms, knees, and shins on the ball, as shown in the photo. At first you might keep one foot on the floor. As you become more experienced, try lifting both feet for short periods of time. This is challenging, but don't get discouraged. The more you try it, the longer you'll be able to balance. My good friend Susan, who is in her sixties, worked up to two full minutes in no time!

Once you feel comfortable balancing on the ball, you can start to learn the four basic body positions used in nearly all the ball exercises.

For the basic body positions, as well as for most of the exercises in this book, you'll need to maintain a *neutral spine*. In other words, keep your head centered above your shoulders—not tipped up or thrust ahead of your shoulders; keep your shoulders low, not hunched toward your ears; make sure your chest is open and your entire spine is long. To get an idea of what this position feels like, stand with your heels, hips, shoulders, and back of your head against a wall. Then walk a few feet away from the wall. Memorize this sensation. Whenever I suggest that you maintain a neutral spine in an exercise, this is the position you want.

Some Words on Safety

When compared with heavy barbells and dumbbells, the ball workout is one of the safest around. The program includes no heavy equipment.

You don't have to worry about dropping anything on your body or getting caught underneath a heavy barbell. Nevertheless, there are some minor concerns, and you should always keep the following safety pointers in mind.

Know Your Space   Avoid accidentally rolling into a coffee table or whacking your hand or foot on a cabinet. Before you do the first exercise, measure out a workout area that's at least 6 feet by 6 feet. Most living rooms have more than that much space if you move the coffee table off to the side.

Get a Checkup   Before starting the ball program, go to your doctor and get a checkup. If you have high blood pressure, lower back pain, a joint disorder, or are pregnant, review the exercises with your doctor to make sure all of them are safe for you.

Listen to Your Body   You should feel your muscles fatigue as you workout, but you should not feel pain. In particular, watch out for pain around your knees, shoulders, spine, or elbows. If an exercise feels uncomfortable at a joint, modify your performance. Sometimes a slight change in position is all you need to make an uncomfortable exercise comfortable. Always listen to the natural wisdom of your body. If you feel pain from a particular exercise no matter how you tweak it, you may have a unique physiology that may not be suited to that particular movement. You have more than fifty different ball exercises to choose from throughout this book, so you can easily omit one or two and still get a great workout.

Always Look Around   Before you attempt any move that requires you to "travel" with the ball, even a short distance, take a look around. Do you have enough space to complete the move without banging into furniture? Has your dog or toddler left a toy on the floor that will impede your progress or cause you to fall off the ball?

THE INCLINE BRIDGE

You'll use the Incline Bridge to do Chest Presses and Chest Flies, Drop Squats, Abdominal Crunches, and many other exercises.

Sit on the ball. Place your palms on the ball on either side of your buttocks. As you use your hands to steady the ball, walk your feet forward as you bend your knees, and allow your buttocks and lower back to slide down the ball. Lower your buttocks a few inches below the height of your knees so that the ball presses into your lower and midback. Once your are in position, relax your hands toward the floor. To rise, press up through your feet as you walk yourself back to the seated position.

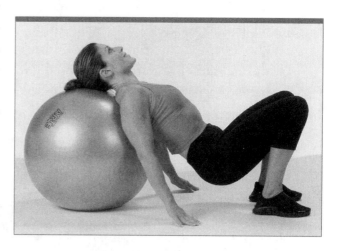

Try walking in and out of this position a few times. If you feel confident with the motion, try doing it with your arms extended from your chest rather than propped against the ball.

THE BRIDGE

You'll use the Bridge for Chest Presses and Chest Flies, Triceps Presses, and Arm Swing Rolls, among other exercises.

Sit on the ball. Walk your feet forward as if you were coming into the Incline Bridge. However, continue to walk your feet away from the ball until only your upper back and shoulders remain in contact with the ball. Press up through your buttocks to form a "bridge," with your knees bent at 90-degree angles. To rise, walk your feet back toward the ball until you return to a seated position. Practice walking in and out of this position a few times.

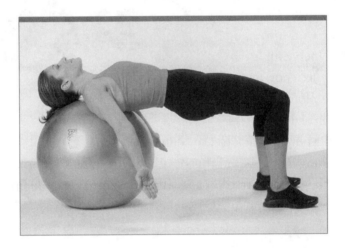

PRONE DRAPE

You'll use the Prone Drape for a variety of exercises, including Upper Back Flies, the Flying Carpet, X Marks the Spot, and many more.

Place the fitness ball in front of you. Kneel on the floor, grasp the ball with both palms and lower your tummy onto the ball. Then take one hand off the ball and place it on the floor. Your palm and the balls of your feet will remain in contact with the floor. To rise, bend your knees until they reach the floor and then push yourself up with your hands.

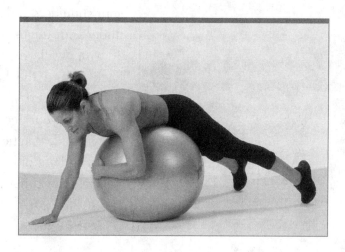

PRONE BRIDGE

You'll use the Prone Bridge to do Push-Ups and Knee Fold-Ups, among other exercises.

Place the fitness ball in front of you. Kneel on the floor, lower your tummy onto the ball, and place your palms flat on the floor, coming into the Prone Drape position. As you walk your hands and upper body forward, allow your torso to slide along the ball until you are bal-

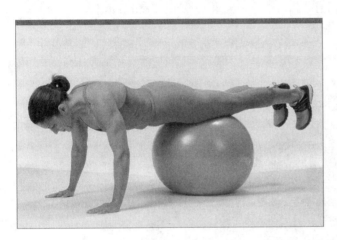

anced in a push-up position, with your hands under your shoulders and the ball under your thighs or shins. To rise, walk your hands back toward the ball and slide backward along the ball until your feet touch the ground. Practice walking in and out of the Prone Bridge a few times.

REVERSE BRIDGE

You'll use the Reverse Bridge to work your legs during Butt Lifts and Hamstring Curls.

   Lie with your back on the mat and your arms at your sides. Place one calf on the ball and then the other calf, keeping your legs bent. Press up through your buttocks and extend and straighten your legs so that the only parts of your body to remain in contact with the mat are your head, arms, and shoulders. Then lower your buttocks back to the mat.

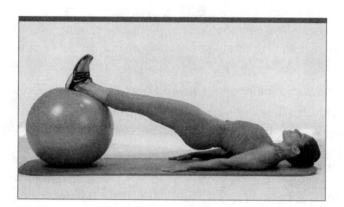

Warm-Up Stretches

Once you feel confident with the basic ball positions, you'll want to move on to warm-up stretches. Before every ball session, warm up your muscles with four important stretches. These stretches have two benefits. First they will help bring circulation to your muscles. Second, they help elongate the muscles to make your subsequent workout more effective. Stretches also feel wonderful!

Spend 60 to 90 seconds on each of the following stretches.

"Good" Fatigue

In all of my ball routines, I specifically prescribe how many repetitions and sets to do for each exercise. However, as you become more proficient with the workouts, I'd like you to listen to your body. It will tell you how many repetitions to do.

Your goal is to work your muscles until fatigue. That means doing an exercise until your muscles are so tired you couldn't possibly perform one more repetition. For each exercise, the last 2 to 3 repetitions should feel difficult. If they don't, you need to either use more weight or increase the number of reps. You may find that you need to do as many as 30 reps to fatigue your muscles. That's fine. In fact, it's desirable, because lower weight and higher reps help you sculpt long, lean muscles. High amounts of weight and low reps, on the other hand, tend to bulk up muscles.

AROUND THE WORLD

When the ball is overhead during this total-body stretch, you target your shoulders, back, and arms. As you lower the ball, you stretch your buttocks and thighs. Around the World is a great warm-up stretch for golfers, because it simulates the motion of a golf swing.

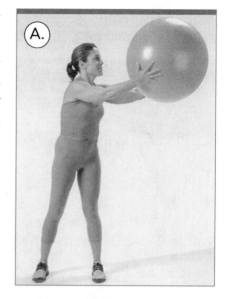

(A.) With your feet a shoulder's width apart, grasp the ball with your palms facing one another. Raise the ball over your left shoulder.

(B.) Slowly lower the ball to the left as you draw an imaginary circle, circling counterclockwise and going down, across your torso, and then up on your right. Start with smaller circles and make them larger as you feel your muscles warm up. Then reverse the motion, circling clockwise.

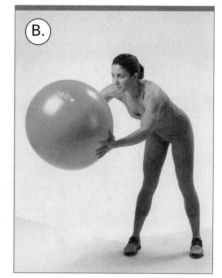

LOW BODY STRETCH

The Low Body Stretch stretches the back of your body, including your lower back and buttocks, as well as the back of your shoulders.

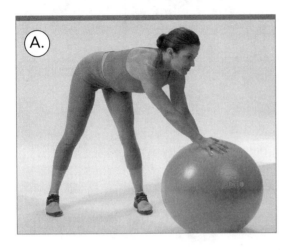

A. With your feet slightly wider than a shoulder's width apart, your knees slightly bent, and the ball in front of your legs, bend forward from your hips and place your palms on top of the ball. Push the ball away from your body until you feel your spine is straight. Bring your right hand over your left as you walk the ball toward your left, feeling a stretch along your outer left back. Hold for 3 to 5 seconds.

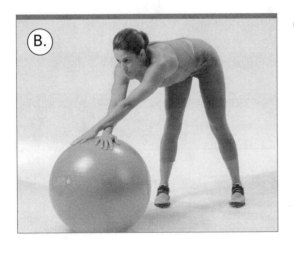

B. Slowly walk the ball back to your right by placing your left hand over your right. You should feel a stretch along your outer left back. Hold for 3 to 5 seconds. Continue rolling the ball back and forth, eventually making larger C shapes with the ball as your body warms up to the stretch.

BUDDHA STRETCH

The Buddha stretches your entire back, particularly your upper back, as well as your hips. This feels wonderful on your spine and is a great stretch to do whenever you've been sitting for a long time and need to work the kinks out of your back.

(A.) Kneel on the mat with the ball about 2 feet in front of you. Reach out and place your palms on top of the ball with your arms completely extended, feeling a stretch in your buttocks and legs.

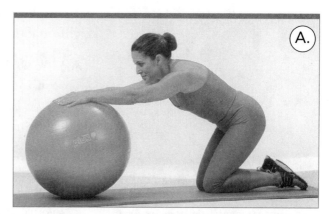

(B.) Bring your buttocks back toward your calves, keeping the ball in place as you do. You should feel a wonderful stretch along your upper back.

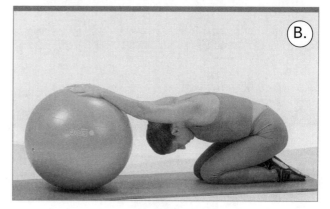

SEATED LEG STRETCH

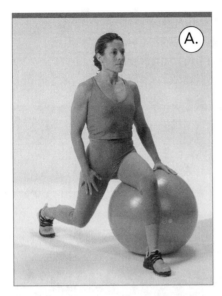

A.

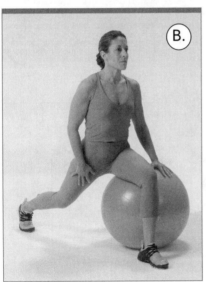

B.

The Seated Leg Stretch stretches the front and back of your thighs, moving the stretch to different areas of your legs as you rock back and forth. It's a great stretch for runners because it relieves tight quadriceps and hip flexor muscles.

A. Sit on the ball in a lunge position with your left thigh pressed into the ball. Extend your right leg behind your torso, with your right knee bent at a 45-degree angle and the weight on the ball of your right foot. Keep your left foot flat on the floor. Place your left palm on the ball for balance.

B. Rock forward by extending through your rear leg and straightening your rear knee slightly. The ball will move forward a couple of inches, moving the stretch up the front of your rear thigh. Continue slowly rocking back and forth for 45 seconds and then switch legs.

You're Making Progress

Some women can complete their first ball routine on the same day they learn the get-acquainted exercises and stretches. Others may still feel awkward on the ball. If you are in the latter group, continue to experiment with the basic ball positions, stretches, and balances until you feel more coordinated. Don't feel rushed. If your first session or two takes longer than 30 minutes, that's fine. Simply balancing on the ball and learning the basic positions still gives your entire body a great workout.

Questions and Answers

Here are the most frequently asked questions about the ball program, along with my answers.

Q. *I started working out with 2.2-pound heavy balls. Now that I can do more than 15 repetitions for each exercise, I bought a set of heavier balls. However, I experience trouble holding these balls. Why do I keep dropping them?*

A. Most women's hands are too small to palm a ball larger than 2.2 pounds. You can use heavier balls for some moves that require a palms-up position but probably not for moves that require the palms to be down.

Continue to use your lighter set of balls and increase the reps beyond 15. You might be able to do as many as 35 to 45 reps before you experience muscle fatigue. Doing this many reps will help you increase your strength and endurance without building bulk.

Q. *I have a bad back. Is it safe for me to do the ball workout?*

A. Fitness balls are great for people with back problems because the ball can support your lower back while you do the moves.

In fact, physical therapists often incorporate fitness balls into back pain rehabilitation programs.

However, some movements do put strain on your lower back. For instance, in the abdominal crunch, less of your back stays in contact with the ball as you lengthen your torso away from it. For this reason you may want to steer clear of crunches and other moves that don't support your back.

Listen to your body as you do your program. If an exercise feels uncomfortable, don't do it. It's worth repeating: Get yourself cleared by a physician before starting the program. Your doctor should look at the exercises and advise you which ones will work for you and which ones will not.

I'm happy to tell you that many people with back pain tell me that their problems subside after a few weeks on the ball program. As their abdominal and back strength increases, their pain and discomfort decrease, and their posture improves.

Q. *Can I get hurt if I fall off my ball?*

A. Working out on a fitness ball is much safer than working out with dumbbells, barbells, and a weight bench, because you have no heavy equipment that can fall on your feet or trap you.

To build your confidence, and thus your balance, go back to the get-acquainted exercises earlier in this chapter. Also, exercise in a safe area, away from sharp objects, table edges, and so on. When you sit on the ball or experiment with different positions, start with your feet against the wall for stability. Planting your feet far apart—wider than a shoulder's width—also provides more stability, whereas bringing your feet closer together gives less stability and makes the moves more challenging.

Q. *I'm more than 100 pounds overweight. Will I crush the fitness ball?*

A. No, you won't. The Gymnic balls, in particular, are designed to withstand more than 600 pounds of pressure. Gymnic also makes a burst-resistant ball. That means if the ball gets punctured, it will lose pressure very slowly, so you won't come crashing to the floor.

Q. *I have small children. Is it safe to do my workout with them in the room?*

A. I encourage you to allow your children to watch you work out. This will plant the seed in their brains that fitness is fun.

That said, remember that toddlers are always on the move. Your toddler may push you or leave a toy nearby that could cause you to stumble and lose your balance.

This doesn't mean you must ban your child from the room when you work out. One option is to talk with other mothers of young children in the neighborhood and try organizing a ball session. As you do one exercise, your friend watches the children. Then switch off so you keep an eye on the toddlers as your friend does her exercise.

If you have to, you can also join a gym that offers daycare. Although the ball program is ideal for home use, you will find that many gyms now offer ball classes. Going to the gym may also give you more ideas and will certainly make your ball session more social.

Finally, consider putting your children in a cordoned-off area or playpen in the room where you are exercising. You can keep an eye on them, and they can't get loose and suddenly cause you to topple.

Q. *My dog seems jealous of my exercise ball. Whenever I try my workout, he pokes me with his nose or paws. What should I do?*

A. I understand your concern. I have two miniature Dachshunds. One of them likes to wedge tiny dog toys under my ball, causing me to lose my balance.

The best strategy is to keep your dogs out of the room while you work out. I put up a kids' guard gate when I exercise. At first the dogs didn't like it and whined at me from the other side of the gate. But eventually they got used to it. I play with them for 5 or 10 minutes after each workout, so they now know that after my workout comes playtime.

You also might try working out during a time of day when your dog is really mellow. Also, try making a "shaky can." Fill an old aluminum soda can with small rocks and tape the opening closed. Then shake the can at your dog and firmly say no whenever he or she comes near you or the ball.

Finally, if you own a large-breed dog, make sure your dog knows that the ball is yours, not his. Your dog's teeth can puncture the ball, so if your pet continues to treat the ball as a toy, store the ball in a safe, out-of-the-way location.

Q. *I want a flat tummy fast. Will working my abs every day help me achieve faster results?*

A. Yes, you can work your abs every day but not for the reason many people think. Your abdominal area is composed of numerous different muscles, and different abdominal exercises target each muscle differently. Try focusing on abdominal crunches one day so that you tire out the front of your abdomen. The next day, do oblique twists to fatigue the sides of your abdomen. Keep in mind that every muscle in your body needs about 48 hours of rest between workouts to repair small muscle tears and gain strength. Muscle soreness is an indication that your abs have not recovered from your last workout. If one part of your abdomen feels sore, don't work that area again until it fully recovers.

Q. *I want to lose weight—yesterday! If I work out on the ball every day, will I achieve faster results?*

A. No. In fact, you'll slow your results. Your body needs 48 hours of rest between workouts to build muscle. If you do your workout every day, you don't give your body enough time to build and repair muscle, and your muscles will become weaker rather than stronger. Stick to three-day-a-week strength workouts, as I suggest in all of my programs. If you'd like to exercise on the alternate days, go

Hitting the Spot

Many women want to tone just one spot on their body. Rather than do a total body strengthening program, they want to work their hips or thighs or abs exclusively. Unfortunately, this type of "spot reducing" doesn't work. When you exercise and build muscle, your body draws energy from fat cells throughout your body to fuel the muscle that's working.

Working your entire body creates a sleeker, leaner body, improving your overall appearance. The total program also boosts your metabolism, aiding your weight-loss efforts. That's why every routine in this book includes exercises for all of the major muscle groups, including the biceps, triceps, core, abs, upper back, lower back, shoulders, chest, and legs.

for a power walk, jog, or do some other form of aerobic exercise. This will help you burn off extra calories while allowing your muscles to recover from the ball sessions.

Q. *I need to work out every single day. I'm worried if I skip a day, I'll never work out again. What should I do?*

A. As I just mentioned, working the same muscles every single day doesn't give them enough time to recover between efforts. However, you can work *alternate* muscles and still achieve results. If you feel you need to work out every day, try working your upper body on Monday, Wednesday, and Friday and your lower body on Tuesday, Thursday, and Saturday. Or, you might alternate your ball workout days with cardiovascular workout days.

Be aware that your mind may need an occasional break from working out. Once in a while, treat yourself to a day at the park or some other low-key activity that you find enjoyable.

Q. *Where can I buy a ball?*

A. Just about every sporting goods store sells fitness balls. You can also buy one online (www.balldynamics.com) or by phone (800-752-2255).

Q. *What's the difference between a heavy ball and a medicine ball?*

A. Medicine balls are the basketball-sized weighted balls used to help train boxers and wrestlers. The heavy balls for ball exercises are small, handheld weighted balls. It's confusing because the two terms have become interchangeable in recent years.

Q. *I already have a set of dumbbells. Do I have to buy the heavy balls?*

A. Heavy balls are just one method for adding resistance during your exercise sessions. I like them the best, but you certainly can use other forms like dumbbells or resistance bands (surgical tubing).

Q. *Do I need someone to spot me for the ball exercises?*

A. Getting used to the ball is really fun, and you can do it without someone spotting you. Just get a ball, put it in your TV room, and practice sitting on it, wiggling around on it, and enjoying yourself. Get used to the ball first before trying the ball program.

Q. *How do I pump up my ball? Does it need a special pump?*

A. The ball will come with a plug and an adaptor. If the plug comes already inserted, remove it. Then lay the ball on a flat surface and smooth out the folds. Next, attach the adaptor to a bike pump or compressor and inflate the ball until it is firm but not completely full. You should be able to press into the ball and have it give about two inches. Because the ball may stretch slightly overnight, you may need to add more air after about 24 hours.

You can purchase a pump specially made for the ball from www .balldynamics.com. Called the "Faster Blaster," this pump requires no adaptor. It also fits in a suitcase, so you can travel with the ball, like I do.

Q. *I'm very athletic. How can I combine my ball program with my other fitness pursuits?*

A. The ball workout greatly helps all athletes, from runners to tennis players to swimmers, by improving balance and coordination as well as muscle strength and endurance. Substitute the ball workout for any traditional strength training with weights, doing the ball workout two to three times a week. During your competitive season, scale back the ball sessions to just two sessions a week. During your off season, spend more time on the ball as you spend less time training competitively.

Q. *What's the difference between my abs and my core?*

A. Your core refers to all of the muscles in your torso that form the center of your body, including your abdominal muscles, back muscles, and the obliques that form your sides. A strong core supports your spine, preventing back pain. It also helps improve your posture. Your core is also your power center. You'll find that strong, coordinated core muscles make you feel stronger and more balanced during everyday activities. You'll climb stairs more easily, walk with more vigor, and generally feel more powerful in everything you do.

Your abs refer to the three muscles that form your abdomen: your rectus abdominus along the front of your abdomen, your obliques along the sides of your abdomen, and your transverse abdominus, a deep abdominal muscle that sits beneath the rectus abdominus.

Now that you have your equipment and you know the basic ball positions and safety tips, you're ready to start your first workout. Remember: Be patient about your abilities. You can do it! So, let's get started.

2

best ball exercises for a beautiful body

Target your arms, abs, back, shoulders, thighs,
and butt in less than 30 minutes a session

Not long after I discovered the benefits of fitness balls for myself, I began designing workouts for just about every friend, acquaintance, and colleague I knew.

During a typical "training session," I excitedly began showing these women exercise after exercise after exercise. Many of my friends were too nice to tell me that I was overwhelming them with too much information. Finally, my good friend and colleague Kris Clark, a nutrition expert at Penn State, told me bluntly: "I only want ten exercises. I can't remember any more than that."

Her comment stayed in my mind as I designed the workouts for this book. I realized that if Kris—who works at fitness every day—didn't want to learn more than ten exercises at once, then most of you probably feel the same.

That's why I worked hard to design a simple yet effective fitness ball program. Though I've included thirty exercises in the six-week schedule, you only need to learn ten of them during any given week.

In the following pages, you'll find three different workouts that include exercises for each of ten main body areas:

1. Abs
2. Back (Upper)
3. Back (Lower)
4. Biceps
5. Chest
6. Core
7. Legs (Thighs)
8. Legs (Butt and Calves)
9. Shoulders
10. Triceps

As I mentioned in chapter 1, working all of these areas helps tone and strengthen your entire body. The three routines will help you build calorie-hungry muscle, important for revving up your metabolism. They will also effectively tone common trouble spots such as the abs, buttocks, and thighs.

During week 1, you'll learn your first ball routine, and you will stick with it through week 2. For weeks 1 and 2, you'll do the following simple yet effective exercises:

Classic Crunches

Upper Torso Lift

Kneeling Back Flies

Preacher Ball Curls

Push-Ups

Knee Fold-Ups

Hamstring Curls

Butt Lift

Push-Offs

Triceps Ball Press

For each workout, start with the four stretches described in chapter 1. Then move into your exercises, doing two sets of 10 to 15 repetitions of each exercise. Between sets and between each exercise, rest for 90 seconds. Perform each exercise slowly, counting from one-one-thousand to four-one-thousand as you complete a movement. Also, try to synchronize your movement with your breathing, exhaling as you complete the hard part of the exercise (such as pressing up during a push-up) and inhaling as you complete the easier part of the exercise (such as lowering during a push-up.)

Complete your workout three times a week.

For weeks 3 and 4, you'll learn the following ten exercises, all of them slightly more challenging than the exercises for weeks 1 and 2:

Ball Crunches

X Marks the Spot

Stomach Back Flies

Bridge-Back Curls

Chest Flies

Kneeling Layouts

Drop Squats

Calf Raises

Right-Angle Lateral Lifts

Bridge Triceps Press

Why change the exercises? Research shows that variety helps keep us motivated. Also, as our bodies become accustomed to each new movement, they perform it more efficiently, lowering calorie burn during exercise. Periodically switching the types of exercises we perform maximizes calorie burn while increasing muscle growth.

However, if you'd rather stick with the same set of ten exercises, that's okay. Just know that your goals may take longer to achieve.

Continue with two sets of 10 to 15 repetitions of each exercise. By week 3 you may be able to cut your rest between sets and exercises to only 60 seconds. However, if you struggle to do the next exercise, keep your rest time at 90 seconds. Complete your workout three times a week.

For weeks 5 and 6, you'll change your routine again, this time doing the following slightly more challenging exercise sequence:

Side-Ups

Standing Torso Twist

Off-the-Ball Back Flies

Off-the-Ball Curls

Chest-Press Incline

Arm-Swing Rolls

Thigh Buster

Atlas Lunge

Flying Carpet

Triceps Extension

Continue with two sets of 10 to 15 repetitions of each exercise. By week 5 you may feel that you are able to lower your rest time between exercises and sets to 30 seconds. However, if you don't feel sufficiently rested during the next set or exercise, go back to resting for a longer period of time. Complete your workout three times a week.

What happens after week 6? You have a number of options. You can continue to switch your exercises every two weeks, starting with the week 1 workouts and progressing to the week 6 workouts. You can also add variety by doing your exercises in reverse order, starting with the triceps extension and finishing with the side-ups. If you feel you are ready for a greater challenge, try the advanced moves in chapter 3, and if you want even greater results, try my six-week body makeover described in part 2.

Are you ready to get started? Then let's go.

Weeks 1 and 2

Abdominals

CLASSIC CRUNCHES

As with regular crunches done on an exercise mat, Classic Crunches specifically target the top section of your rectus abdominus, or the front of your abdomen above your navel. However, when crunches are done on the ball rather than on a mat, you must use numerous smaller muscles along your sides and even in your buttocks, thighs, and calves to maintain your balance.

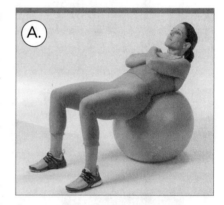

(A.) Sit on the ball with your feet flat on the floor and a shoulder's distance apart. Slide down on the ball until it supports your lower and midback. Relax your neck and make sure your chin is a fist's distance away from your chest. Fold your arms across your chest.

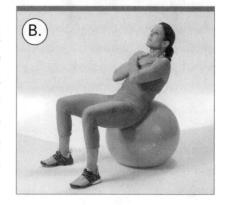

(B.) Contract your abs as you exhale and crunch up, bringing your ribs closer to your hips. Inhale as you slowly lower. Remember to keep your neck long and relaxed. As you crunch, try not to tense your neck muscles by jutting your head forward over your shoulders or by bringing your chin toward your chest. I've found that pressing the tip of my tongue against the roof of my mouth prevents me from craning my neck forward. Repeat 10 to 15 times.

Ball Basics

- The closer your feet are to each other, the tougher your balancing act. If you experience trouble balancing, place your feet wider than a shoulder's distance apart. If you find the exercise too easy, bring your feet and knees closer together.

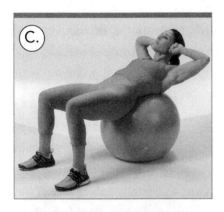

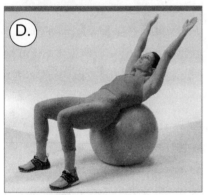

- For an extra challenge, change your hand position. Try doing the crunch with your fists just in front of your ears, your elbows out to your sides, and your chest open, as shown in photo C. If you need an even greater challenge, try the crunch with your arms extended overhead, as shown in photo D.

- How much of your back you rest against the ball determines the difficulty of the exercise. The more you let the ball support your back, the less challenging the move.

Back (Lower)

UPPER TORSO LIFT

The Upper Torso Lift targets the lower back and works the muscles that line your spine, helping improve your posture. It also works your legs and buttocks.

A. Lie in a prone position with your waist and tummy on the ball and your legs extended. Place the balls of your feet on the floor, with your right leg pointing at 4 o'clock and your left at 8 o'clock. Mold your body to the ball and place your fists by your ears.

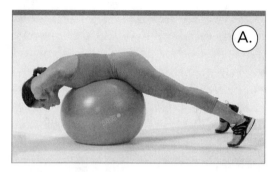

B. Extend up as you exhale, bringing your shoulders toward the ceiling and straightening your spine. Stop once your back is flat. Lower as you inhale. Repeat 10 to 15 times.

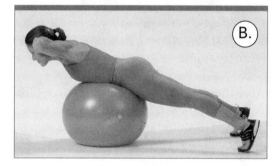

Ball Basics

- Try not to hyperextend your back in this exercise by raising your shoulders higher than your buttocks.

- You can change your arm position to increase the challenge of this exercise. Rather than keeping your fists by your ears, try doing the exercise with your arms extended in front, as shown in photo C. To increase the challenge even more, try the torso lift while holding a heavy ball in each hand.

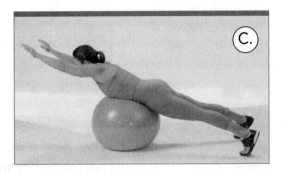

- The closer your feet are to one another, the tougher your balancing act.

Back (Upper)

KNEELING BACK FLIES

Have you ever felt a pain right between your shoulder blades? This exercise targets that area and will help you carry a backpack pain-free.

(A.) Lie in a prone position with your chest on the ball and your knees, shins, and feet against the mat. Grasp a pair of heavy balls. Extend your arms and place your right arm at 3 o'clock and your left at 9 o'clock. Lift the balls 2 inches off the floor.

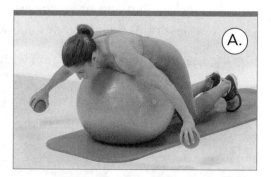

(B.) Exhale as you raise the balls to torso level, drawing your shoulder blades closer together as you do so. Inhale as you lower. Repeat 10 to 15 times.

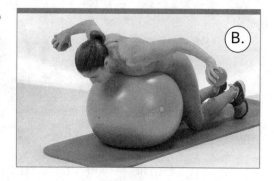

Ball Basics

- Never lock your joints. Though your arms are extended to your sides during this exercise, you should keep a slight bend in your elbows at all times.

- You can modify this exercise simply by changing your arm position. Holding your arms at 2 and 10 o'clock or at 11 and 1 o'clock will slightly change the target area along the back of your shoulders.

Biceps

PREACHER BALL CURLS

The first in this series of upper arm exercises offers you the most stability, because you will be pressing your upper arms against the ball. In weeks 2 and 3, your biceps exercises will become progressively harder as less of your body comes in contact with the ball.

(A.) Lie in a prone position with your tummy on the ball. Extend your legs, keeping a slight bend in your knees and placing the balls of your feet against the floor. Grasp a heavy ball in each hand. Bend your arms and press the backs of your upper arms and elbows into the ball.

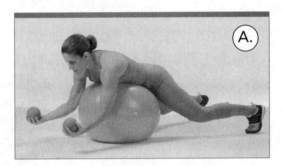

(B.) Exhale as you slowly curl your hands toward your shoulders—you should take at least 4 seconds to raise your hands to shoulder level. Inhale as you lower slowly. Repeat 10 to 15 times.

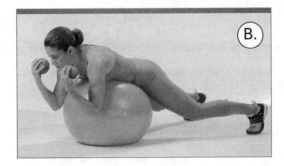

Ball Basics

- If you experience difficultly remaining balanced, use a mat and kneel so that your knees touch the mat.

- For variety, try alternating arms, curling first with your left arm, lowering, and then curling with your right.

- For an additional challenge, try doing the exercise with your upper arms and elbows a few inches in front of the ball.

Chest

PUSH-UPS

This variation on traditional military push-ups does much more than target your chest muscles. Your abdominals and buttocks also work hard as you stay balanced on the ball.

(A.) Lie in a prone position with your belly on the ball. Scoot forward along the ball until you can place your palms on the floor directly under your shoulders. Keep your balance by pressing your thighs against the ball. Place your feet in a relaxed and neutral position—neither hyperflexed nor pointed—with your toes pointing down.

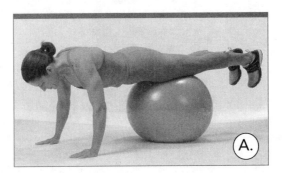

(B.) Inhale as you lower your chest to the floor by bending your elbows. Stop once your chin is even with the bend in your elbows. Exhale as you press back to the starting position. Repeat 10 to 15 times.

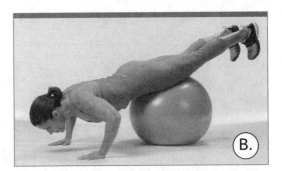

Ball Basics

- You can increase the difficulty of this exercise by scooting forward so that only your lower legs or your feet rest against the ball (see photo C). First, try the move with your shins against the ball. Then try it with the tops of your feet against the ball. Finally, try it with only your toes on the ball.

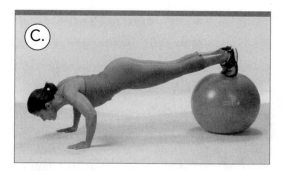

- Keep your back flat throughout the exercise. Don't allow your hips to sink down, because then your lower back will arch.

Core

KNEE FOLD-UPS

Knee Fold-Ups are great for your entire core—your abs, buttocks, sides, and back. They also test your coordination and balance, as well as work your chest.

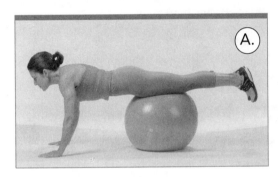

A. Place the fitness ball in front of your body. Kneel on the floor, lower your tummy onto the ball, and place your palms flat on the floor. Walk your hands and upper body forward. Your torso will slide along the ball until you are balanced in a push-up position, with your hands under your shoulders and the ball under your thighs.

B. As you exhale, press your shins into the ball and draw them forward, bending your knees and bringing your legs and the ball under your torso. Uncoil and inhale as you press the ball back out to the starting position. Repeat 10 to 15 times.

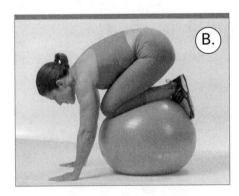

Ball Basics

- You can increase the challenge of this exercise by starting with the ball under your shins.

- You can increase the challenge even more by starting with the ball under the balls of your feet. However, doing so causes the motion of the exercise to change somewhat. Instead of bending your knees, pull the ball forward and bring your body into a jackknife or V-shape position, with your buttocks above your shoulders and your legs extended.

Legs (Thighs)

HAMSTRING CURLS

Forget hamstring curls on the machine at the gym or even curls on a mat with ankle weights. You haven't toned your hamstrings until you've tried Hamstring Curls on the ball. This move effectively targets the muscles along the backs of your thighs, as well as your abs, buttocks, and lower back. Don't be surprised if you immediately feel the burn on your first few repetitions.

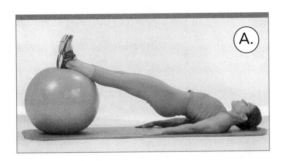

A. Lie with your back on the mat. Extend your legs and place the backs of your heels on the fitness ball. Rest your arms on the floor by your sides. Press your heels into the ball to lift your buttocks, forming a straight line from your feet to your shoulders. Once you're in position, only the backs of your shoulders and head should rest against the mat.

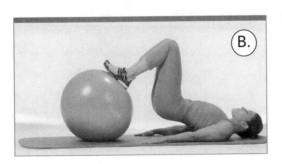

B. As you exhale, bend your knees, press your heels into the ball, and pull it in toward your buttocks. Then inhale as you extend your legs and press the ball back out to the starting position. Repeat 10 to 15 times.

Ball Basics

- Keep your buttocks pressed up and your back flat throughout the exercise; try not to let your buttocks sink toward the floor.

- The closer you place your arms to your body, the more challenging the exercise.

- For a greater challenge, try lifting your forearms up and pointing your fingers toward the ceiling. For an even greater challenge, cross your arms over your chest.

Legs (Butt/Calves)

BUTT LIFT

The Butt Lift targets the piece of fat that tends to hang below the bottom of a bathing suit. This move also works your thighs, back, and abs to help you balance on the ball.

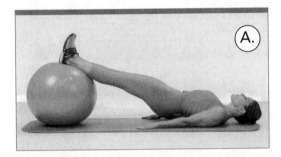

A. Lie on your back with your legs extended and heels pressed into the top of the ball. Rest your arms by your sides. Tighten your abs as you lift your buttocks a couple of inches off the mat.

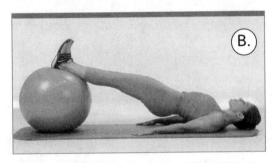

B. Exhale as you press your hips up, creating a straight line from your heels to your shoulders. Inhale as you lower to the starting position. Repeat 10 to 15 times.

Ball Basics

- Try not to rest your buttocks on the mat between repetitions.

- The closer you place your arms to your body, the more challenging the exercise.

- For a greater challenge, try lifting your forearms up and pointing your fingers toward the ceiling. For an even greater challenge, cross your arms over your chest.

Shoulders

PUSH-OFFS

Push-Offs aren't the prettiest exercise in the world, but they may be the most fun. In addition to working your shoulders, the pressing motion of this exercise targets your chest and buttocks.

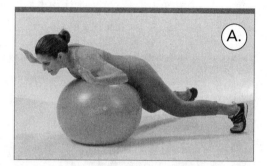

(A.) Lie in a prone position with your tummy on the ball, your knees bent, and the balls of your feet on the floor. Bend your arms and hold them out to your sides, palms facing forward.

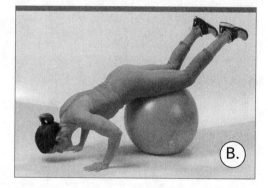

(B.) As if you were a frog jumping through the air, push off with your feet as you inhale. The movement of your torso will roll the ball forward. Dive forward and land on your palms with your feet in the air, keeping your abdomen on the ball. Exhale as you push off with your hands and land in the starting position. Repeat 10 to 15 times.

Ball Basics

- Don't allow your head to touch the floor.

- Keep your head in line with your back. Avoid looking upward and hyperextending your neck.

- Be sure to keep your abdomen on the ball when you push off.

- This should be a controlled movement throughout.

Triceps

TRICEPS BALL PRESS

If you've ever tried "dips" either on a bench or on a dip bar, you'll love the Triceps Ball Press. Staying balanced on the ball will use just about every muscle in your body as you constantly adjust and readjust. If you complete 10 reps without falling off, give yourself a confident pat on the back for a job well done.

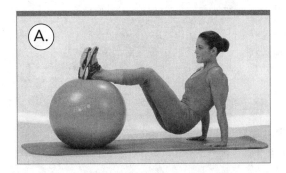

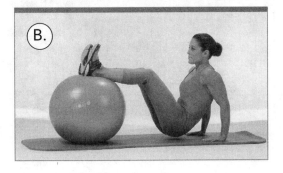

A. Sit on the mat with your hands behind your buttocks on either side of your hips. Your fingertips should be pointing toward the ball in front of you. Place your calves on top of the fitness ball with your legs bent. Press through the palms of your hands and lift your buttocks off the mat as you straighten your elbows.

B. Inhale as you lower your torso and bend your elbows. Don't allow your buttocks to touch the floor. Exhale as you rise. Repeat 10 to 15 times.

Ball Basics

- If you find this exercise too difficult, place more of your legs against the ball.

- To increase the challenge, place only the backs of your heels on the ball. You can also try it with only one leg on the ball and the other elevated a couple of inches above the ball.

Weeks 3 and 4

Abductionals

Abdominals

BALL CRUNCHES

The Ball Crunch combines the Classic Crunch from weeks 1 and 2 with a reverse crunch. It targets not only the top of your rectus abdominus but also the bottom part below the navel. It's a great time-saving exercise, particularly for women who notice a bulge below the belly button.

(A.) Lie on your back. Place the ball between your knees and hug it with your legs. Place your fingertips lightly along the back of your skull, with your elbows bent and out to the sides.

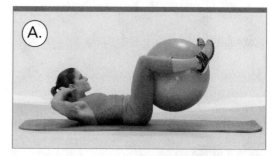

(B.) Lift your chest as you simultaneously exhale and curl your tailbone up, bringing your buttocks and shoulders off the mat like a clam closing its shell. Remember to keep your chin at least a fist's distance away from your chest. Lower as you inhale. Repeat 10 to 15 times.

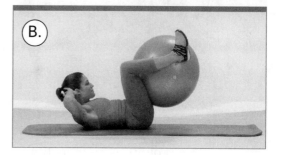

Ball Basics

• Keep a fist's distance between your chin and chest as you crunch.

• Keep your elbows out to your sides as you crunch. If you can see your elbows, they are too far forward.

Back (Lower)

X MARKS THE SPOT

I love X Marks the Spot because it helps tone the lower back as well as most of the back side of the body, particularly the buttocks.

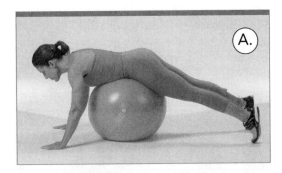

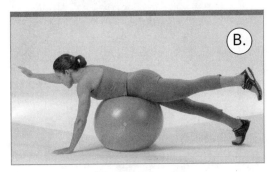

A. Lie in a prone position with your tummy on the ball. Place your feet on the floor, with your right leg pointing at 4 o'clock and your left at 8 o'clock. Place your hands on the floor, with your right hand at 2 o'clock and your left at 11 o'clock. Your body will form an X shape if seen from above.

B. Exhale and simultaneously lift your right arm and your left leg. Inhale and lower your arm and leg. Exhale and repeat with your left arm and right leg. Continue switching back and forth for 10 to 15 repetitions. (Lifting your right arm and left leg and then your left arm and right leg counts as one repetition.)

Ball Basics

- As you lift your opposite arm and leg, keep your glutes tight.

- When in the up position, don't hyperextend. Raise your arm and leg only as high as your torso.

Back (Upper)

STOMACH BACK FLIES

Stomach Back Flies look similar to the Kneeling Back Flies from weeks 1 and 2. The difference is, in this exercise more of your body is off the ball, making it tougher to keep your balance and requiring you to work more muscles.

A. Lie in a prone position with your tummy and ribs on the ball and your legs extended behind you, with your right leg pointing at 4 o'clock and your left at 8 o'clock. Place only the balls of your feet against the floor. Hold a pair of heavy balls in each hand, and position your right arm at 3 o'clock and your left at 9 o'clock. Lift the balls 2 inches off the floor, with your thumbs facing inward and fingertips pointed downward.

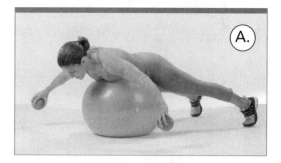

B. Exhale and raise the balls, bringing your shoulder blades toward each other as you lift your elbows up and in, in a small arc. Inhale and lower.

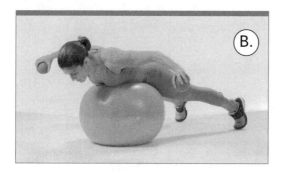

Ball Basics

- Keep your head and neck in a neutral, natural position throughout the movement.

- Keep your shoulder blades pressed down your back (not hunched toward your ears).

Biceps

BRIDGE-BACK CURLS

Bridge-Back Curls offer yet another total body exercise. Although they specifically target your biceps as you raise and lower the heavy ball, they also require you to use your abdominal, buttocks, and thigh muscles to keep your body pressed against the ball.

A. Lie on the ball in a modified bridge position, with your upper back pressed against the ball, your knees bent, and your feet flat on the floor. Grasp a heavy ball in each hand with your palms facing up and your hands at hip level. Exhale and curl your left hand toward your left shoulder.

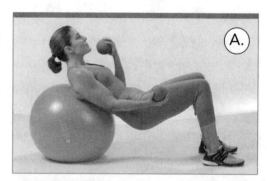

B. As you inhale, slowly lower your left hand and raise your right hand toward your right shoulder. Then exhale and lower your right hand as you raise your left. Continue alternating for 10 to 15 repetitions.

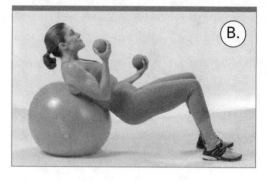

Ball Basics

- Keep your glutes, hamstrings, and abs tight throughout the exercise.

Chest

CHEST FLIES

Chest Flies target the sides of the chest, particularly the troublesome piece of flab near the armpit that tends to stick out of a bathing suit top. You'll also work your thighs, abs, and buttocks as you maintain your balance against the ball.

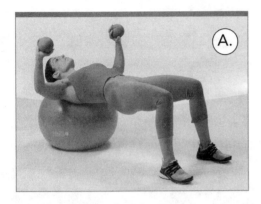

A. Lie in a bridge position with your upper back on the ball, your knees bent, and your feet flat on the floor. Hold a pair of heavy balls in each hand with your elbows bent and arms out to your sides at shoulder level.

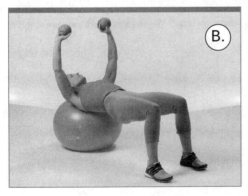

B. Exhale and press the balls toward one another in a large arcing motion, bringing your chest muscles closer together. Inhale and lower. Repeat 10 to 15 times.

Ball Basics

• Don't allow your elbows to go below your shoulders.

• Keep your legs, abs, and glutes tight in a tabletop shape throughout the exercise; don't allow your glutes to sink down.

Core

KNEELING LAYOUTS

Great for your entire abdominal region, Kneeling Layouts are also downright fun. Layouts are a great exercise to try with your children.

(A.) Kneel on the mat with the ball in front of you, close to your torso. Clasp your hands together in a modified prayer position, pressing the bottoms of your hands and forearms against the ball. Balance on your knees by lifting your feet and calves off the exercise mat.

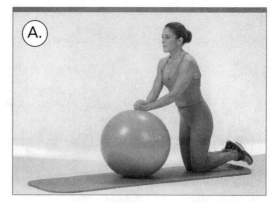

(B.) As you exhale, press into the ball with your hands and forearms and roll the ball forward. Your knees will stay put, but your shins and feet will rise higher off the mat. Inhale as you return to the starting position. Repeat 10 to 15 times.

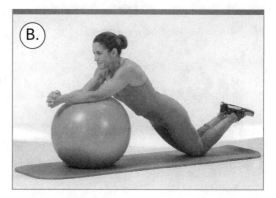

Ball Basics

- As you roll forward, keep your back flat.

- The farther you are from the ball, the more challenging the exercise.

- For a greater challenge, try the exercise with your palms pressed flat against the top or the sides of the ball.

Legs (Thighs)

DROP SQUATS

Squats work your entire backside, as well as your abs. The problem with doing traditional squats from a standing position, however, is that many women find they experience knee and back pain. Doing them against the ball eliminates pain and magnifies the benefits.

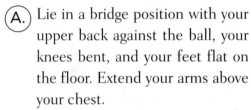

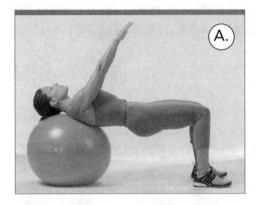

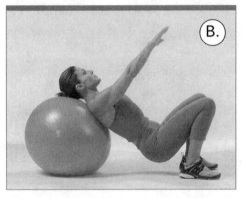

A. Lie in a bridge position with your upper back against the ball, your knees bent, and your feet flat on the floor. Extend your arms above your chest.

B. Inhale and squat down as you bend your knees and sink your buttocks toward the floor. Allow the ball to roll as your back moves downward. Exhale and press back up to the starting position. Repeat 10 to 15 times.

Ball Basics

- To make the move harder, cross your arms over your chest.

- Keep your abs tight throughout the exercise.

Legs (Butt/Calves)

CALF RAISES

Many women focus on only the most troublesome areas of the legs—the butt and thighs—and ignore their calves. Yet, strong, shapely calves will help you perform better in just about every fitness pursuit. They also mean your legs look terrific in Capri-style pants.

(A.) Stand a few feet away from a wall, with your fitness ball between your tummy and the wall. Lean forward into the ball so that your body forms a straight line from your heels to your head.

(B.) Exhale and rise onto the balls of your feet. Inhale and lower. Repeat 10 to 15 times.

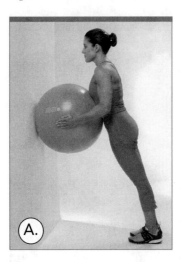 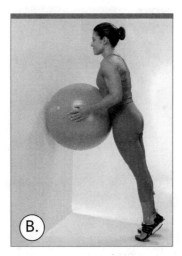

Ball Basics

- Keep your back flat throughout the exercise.

- Avoid hyperextending your knees. Keep them slightly bent, not locked.

Shoulders

RIGHT-ANGLE LATERAL LIFTS

In traditional lateral lifts you raise both arms out to your sides, and this targets your shoulders just fine. However, I find that raising the arms in an alternating right angle makes the exercise feel more fluid.

(A.) Sit on the fitness ball with your knees bent and feet flat on the floor. Hold a heavy ball in each hand and keep your hands at your sides. Exhale as you simultaneously lift your right arm in front of your torso and your left arm laterally out to your side, forming a right angle with your arms. Stop once your arms reach shoulder level.

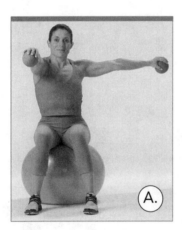 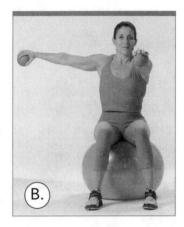

(B.) Inhale and lower your arms. Exhale as you raise your left arm in front of your body and your right arm laterally to the side. Lower and continue alternating for 10 to 15 repetitions.

Ball Basics

- The first few times you do this exercise, you may experience difficulty palming the ball. Do the exercise as many times as you can with your palms facing the floor. If your hands fatigue before your shoulders do, perform the rest of the repetitions with a smaller ball and repeat as many times as you need (as many as 20 to 25 reps) to fatigue your shoulders.

- Don't raise your arms higher than your shoulders.

Triceps

BRIDGE TRICEPS PRESS

In addition to targeting the muscle along the back of your upper arm, the Bridge Triceps Press also works your thighs, buttocks, and abs.

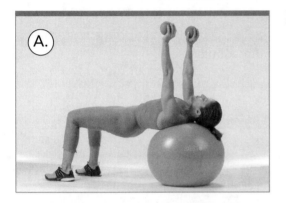

(A.) Lie in a bridge position with your upper back on the ball, your knees bent at 90-degree angles, and your feet flat on the floor. Grasp a heavy ball in each hand and extend your arms at chest level, forming a 90-degree angle between your arms and your chest.

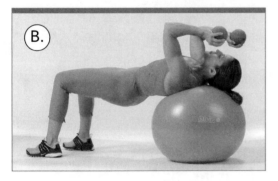

(B.) While keeping your lower arms fixed in position, inhale and lower your hands toward your face. Exhale and press up to the starting position. Repeat 10 to 15 times.

Ball Basics

- When you lower the balls, don't allow them to touch your head.

- Press up through your thighs and buttocks throughout the exercise, keeping your torso in a tight tabletop.

- Keep your upper arms stable and motionless throughout the exercise.

Weeks 5 and 6

Abbdominals

SIDE-UPS

Side-Ups target your obliques (the abdominal muscles that form your waist). This move works particularly well for women who want to tone up those love handles. To balance, you also use numerous muscles throughout your body, including the deep abdominal muscle called the transverse abdominus.

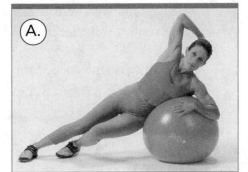

A. Kneel on the floor and position your left hip and side against the ball. Bend your left leg and straighten your right, placing both feet flat on the floor. Bend your right arm and place the palm of your right hand on the back of your head. Bend your left arm and place it on the ball for balance.

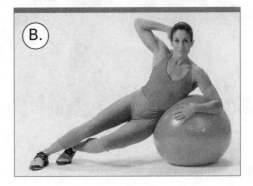

B. Exhale and crunch up, raising your right shoulder and curling your right ribs closer to your right hip. Inhale and lower. Repeat 10 to 15 times, then switch sides.

Ball Basics

- If you experience trouble balancing, place the foot of your extended leg against a wall for leverage.

Back (Lower)

STANDING TORSO TWIST

The lower back exercises you learned in weeks 1 through 4 help your back extend or lift up but not twist. Numerous activities in life, such as reaching to shut off your alarm clock, require you to twist your back. The twisting motion of this exercise will tone the muscles along your spine, your lower back, and your sides and will help create a healthy, pain-free back.

(A.) Stand with your legs a shoulder's width apart. Hold your fitness ball at waist level. Exhale and twist your torso to your left.

(B.) Inhale and slowly bring the ball in a semicircle to the right as you twist your torso. Repeat 10 to 15 times.

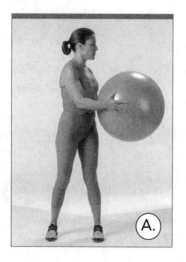 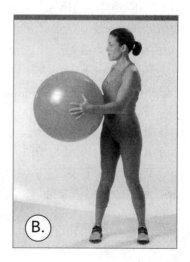

Ball Basics

- Keep both hip bones pointing forward throughout the exercise. Your hips should remain stable and motionless as you twist.

- As you move, keep your abs and your glutes tight.

Back (Upper)

OFF-THE-BALL BACK FLIES

Of all the upper back exercises you learn in this program, Off-the-Ball Back Flies are the toughest. In this exercise, you shift half your torso off the ball, creating a great balancing challenge.

A. Lie in a prone position with your tummy on the ball, similar to Stomach Back Flies. Now, shift your body so that only the right side of your torso remains pressed against the ball. (The left side of your torso hangs over the ball.) Hug the ball with your right

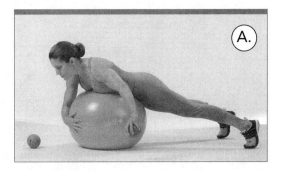

arm and extend your legs so that your right leg points at 4 o'clock and your left at 8 o'clock. Grasp a heavy ball in your left hand and keep your fingers pointing down.

B. Exhale and raise the heavy ball, leading with your elbow slightly bent (not locked) and bringing your left shoulder blade toward your right shoulder blade. You should feel this in your left upper back as well as in your right buttock. Inhale and lower. Repeat 10 to 15 times and then switch sides.

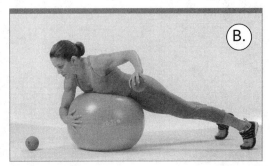

Ball Basics

- Because only part of your torso rests against the ball, this move requires quite a bit of balance. If you find you can't stay balanced, spread your feet wider apart.

- If you seek a greater challenge, try this move with the leg opposite your lifting arm extended and off the floor.

Biceps

OFF-THE-BALL CURLS

As with Off-the-Ball Back Flies, Off-the-Ball Curls test your balancing skills. This exercise requires you to keep most of your body off the ball and makes you use muscles from your head to your toes as you balance.

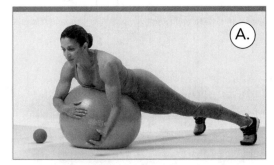

A. Lie prone on the ball. Shift your body so that only the right side of your torso presses against the ball. Extend your legs, pointing your right leg to 4 o'clock and your left to 8 o'clock. Press the balls of your feet into the floor. Hug the ball with your right arm and grasp a heavy ball in your left hand, palm facing up. Press your left elbow into the ball.

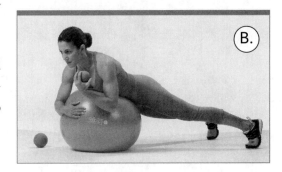

B. Exhale and curl your left hand toward your left shoulder. Inhale and lower. Repeat 10 to 15 times, then switch sides.

Ball Basics

- Because only part of your torso rests against the ball, this move requires quite a bit of balance. If you find you can't stay balanced, spread your feet wider apart.

- Keep your abs tight throughout the exercise.

- If you seek a greater challenge, try this move with the leg opposite your lifting hand extended and off the floor.

Chest

CHEST-PRESS INCLINE

The Chest-Press Incline targets the top of your chest muscles and helps create an illusion of cleavage in women with small breasts. You'll also work your abs, thighs, and buttocks during this exercise.

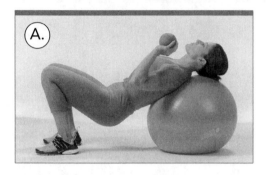

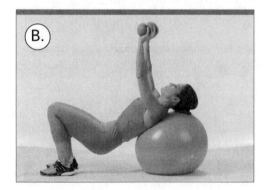

A. Lie in a bridge position with your back against the ball, your knees bent, and your feet flat on the floor. Roll forward on the ball, bringing your buttocks a few inches below the height of your knees.

Grasp a heavy ball in each hand and bend your elbows with palms facing up. Make sure your upper arms are on the same plane as your torso and close to your body.

B. Exhale and press the balls up, straightening your arms above your chest. Inhale and lower. Repeat 10 to 15 times.

Ball Basics

- For an added challenge, roll forward so that less of your upper back is supported by the ball.

- Keep your buttocks and abs tight throughout the exercise.

Core

ARM-SWING ROLLS

Arm-Swing Rolls require slow, controlled movement and mindful attention to balance and coordination.

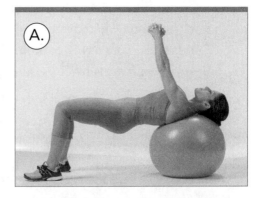

A. Lie in a bridge position with your upper back against the ball. Extend your arms over your chest and clasp your hands together. Press up through your thighs and buttocks so that your body forms a tabletop.

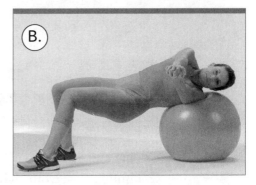

B. Exhale and lower your hands to your left as you roll onto the outside of your left shoulder. Your right shoulder, torso, and buttock will rise up as your left hip lowers. When you are fully in position, your left shoulder blade will not touch the ball. Inhale, return to the starting position, and repeat to your right. Continue switching sides for 10 to 15 repetitions on each side.

Ball Basics

• Keep your buttocks tight throughout the exercise.

• Press up through your butt and thighs to remain firmly in a bridge position as you move from side to side.

Legs (Thighs)

THIGH BUSTER

Thigh Buster does just what the name implies: It tones the outer part of the thigh where women often complain of saddlebags. Because you must use your arms to hold the ball in place, the thigh buster also works your arms (triceps) and shoulders (deltoids).

(A.) Lie on your left side on the mat. Place the fitness ball on top of your right thigh, using your right hand to hold the ball in place. Bend your left arm and prop up your head with your left hand.

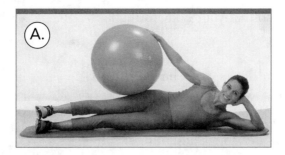

(B.) Exhale and, leading with your right heel, lift your right leg. Continue to use your right hand to hold the ball in place. Inhale and lower. Repeat 10 to 15 times, then switch sides.

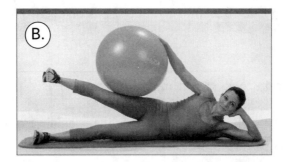

Ball Basics

- To increase the challenge, bend your top leg to form a 90-degree angle and bring it forward so that your top foot is in front of your bottom knee, with the ball balanced on your top outer thigh.

- You can also increase the challenge by applying more hand pressure against the ball.

Legs (Butt/Calves)

ATLAS LUNGE

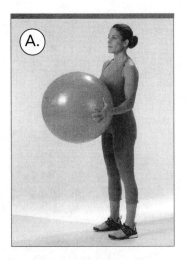

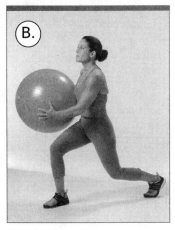

The Atlas Lunge combines the traditional lunge with a twist to work your butt, calves, thighs, abs, and back. Holding the ball also allows you to target your shoulders.

A. Stand with your feet a shoulder's width apart. Hold the ball a few inches in front of your torso at waist level.

B. Inhale and lunge forward with your right leg as you twist your upper body to the right. Make sure you keep your forearms parallel to the floor. Sink down into the lunge, bending your right leg as much as 90 degrees as you extend through your rear leg. Exhale and press back to the starting position. Repeat with your left leg. Continue alternating, totaling 10 to 15 lunges on each leg.

Ball Basics

- Do this move in a slow, controlled motion. Take a small step at first and increase your stepping distance as you become more comfortable.

- The first few times you try this exercise, you may not be fluid in connecting your twist with your lunge. In time, however, you'll learn to work your upper and lower body in one coordinated movement.

- When you lunge forward, don't bend your knee beyond 90 degrees. Your knee should stay above your heel.

Shoulders

FLYING CARPET

The Flying Carpet targets the top
and front of your shoulders, as well
as your lower back.

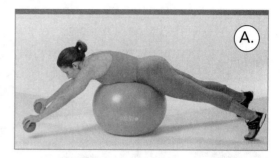

A. Lie prone on the fitness ball
with your legs extended and
the balls of your feet on the
floor. Point your right leg at
4 o'clock and your left at 8
o'clock. Grasp a heavy ball in each hand and extend your arms in
front of you. Lift the heavy balls about an inch from the floor.

B. Exhale and extend your arms up to shoulder level. Then inhale
and lower to the starting position. Repeat 10 to 15 times.

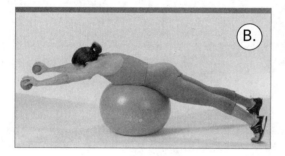

Ball Basics

• Try not to rest the balls on the floor between repetitions.

• Keep your gaze about 3 feet in front of your fitness ball.

• The closer you place your legs to one another, the tougher it is to
balance on the ball.

Triceps

TRICEPS EXTENSION

Unlike the two triceps exercises you learned in weeks 1 through 4, the Triceps Extension works your upper arms in a straightened position, targeting the muscle in a slightly different manner.

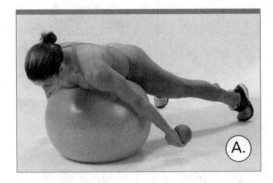

A. Lie prone with your tummy on the fitness ball, your legs extended, and the balls of your feet on the floor. Point your right foot toward 4 o'clock and your left toward 8 o'clock. Grasp a heavy ball in each hand. Extend your arms back along your sides with your knuckles close to the floor.

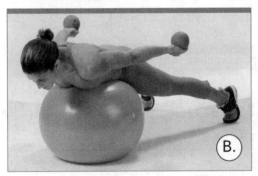

B. Exhale and raise your arms, bringing the heavy balls toward your hips. Inhale and lower. Repeat 10 to 15 times.

Ball Basics

- The closer you bring your legs to one another, the harder it is to stay balanced on the ball.

- Avoid resting your hands and heavy balls on the floor between repetitions.

3

building your confidence

Challenging tips, tricks, and exercises to push your fitness to the next level

Some women have what I like to call "post-traumatic gym-class syndrome." They tell me they have no confidence in their ability to carry out a fitness program because of failed attempts in the past. They say these attempts usually were under the direction of a drill sergeant–type middle or high school physical education teacher.

Such unenlightened teachers made children climb ropes, do push-ups and pull-ups, and run sprints—all with little or no conditioning or preparatory training. Not surprisingly, many girls and young women failed these phys ed classes. They clung to the rope but couldn't climb it. They hung from the pull-up bar but couldn't pull themselves up.

As a result of this poor instruction, these women grew up with the flawed belief that they lacked the genetic wherewithal to perform "advanced" exercises.

This notion is wrong. With proper training, women can perform pull-ups, rope climbs, push-ups, and other tough moves. I'm living proof. When I started pull-ups, my achievement was zero. I went from that to my all time high of 57!

I say all this not because I want you to head for the gym and start doing pull-ups or rope climbs but to convince you that you may be capable of doing more demanding workouts than you think. Every woman's body responds to exercise by growing stronger. What felt awkward and hard two days ago will always feel just a bit easier today.

So challenge yourself.

Being "up" for the challenge will help increase your ball program results. In the beginning of any new fitness program, we all shed extra pounds and improve our strength somewhat easily. It's after we slim down and become stronger that we need to work harder to see results. And, when we do the same moves day after day, we start to get bored. Our results drop off because our muscles have learned to do the exercises by rote, burning fewer calories. Our brains go on strike, and we struggle with ourselves to do our exercises. Soon we may stop doing them altogether.

In my exercise ball program, by challenging yourself with new, more interesting exercises, you surmount those weight-loss plateaus and keep your muscles and brain consistently alert. End result: You always look forward to your workouts, you stick to the program, and your muscles burn more calories during and after each session.

Meeting challenges also builds confidence. I love to see the smiles on women's faces after they've completed their first push-up. Suddenly, they realize that they *can* do it. This is the kind of confidence that carries over beyond your workout. Suddenly, you are taking on challenges at work and in your relationships. Your outlook on life changes. Where once you may have avoided obstacles, now you take them on with vigor.

Challenges help us grow. Without them, we never test our courage, fitness, and confidence. Without them, we never try new things. Without them, life becomes boring.

Challenging yourself is what this chapter is all about. It is not a chapter for beginners on the exercise ball. Before trying the moves in this chapter, you should first spend six weeks doing the exercises in chapter 2.

You know you're ready for a greater challenge when:

- You can easily do 15 repetitions or more of the exercises in chapter 2 without feeling wobbly on the ball.

- You're beginning to feel bored with the exercises in chapter 2.

During your first week with these new exercises, you may be able to do only a few repetitions. That's okay. You can always finish your 30-minute session with a similar exercise from chapter 2. Let's say you complete 3 repetitions of the Torso Lift and Twist on page 82. You can finish up with 10 or more repetitions of the Torso Lift in chapter 2.

Remember: Challenges build confidence!

Confidence Builders

Here are some tips for making your existing program more challenging.

Learn to Vary Your Routine   You can add variety and challenge to your program simply by changing the order of the exercises. Remember, the more variety you give your muscles, the harder they must work to do the exercise and the more entertained your brain feels during your workout. Try to make every workout slightly different. By the end of this chapter, you'll know a total of forty exercises—that's ten new challenging moves from this chapter and thirty from chapter 2. Mix and match exercises from the two chapters and include different exercises in every workout. (See the Muscle Memory chart to learn which muscles are targeted by each exercise.)

Preexhaust Each Muscle Group   Perform two or even three back-to-back exercises for the same muscle group. If you're working your chest, start with the Chest Flies, and then, without resting, move into the Chest Press or the Push-Up. Or, when working your biceps, start with Preacher Ball Curls and move directly into Bridge-Back Curls or Off-the-Ball Curls.

Muscle Memory

Use this chart to create your own customized workouts.

ABS
Classic Crunches (p. 31)
Ball Crunches (p. 47)
Side-Ups (p. 59)
Oblique Twist (p. 78)

BACK (LOWER)
Upper Torso Lift (p. 33)
X Marks the Spot (p. 48)
Standing Torso Twist (p. 60)
Torso Lift and Twist (p. 82)

BACK (UPPER)
Kneeling Back Flies (p. 35)
Stomach Back Flies (p. 49)
Off-the-Ball Back Flies (p. 61)
Alternating Flies (p. 80)

BICEPS
Preacher Ball Curls (p. 36)
Bridge-Back Curls (p. 51)
Off-the-Ball Curls (p. 63)
Off-the-Ball Curls (on one leg)
   (p. 83)

CHEST
Push-Ups (p. 38)
Chest Flies (p. 52)
Chest-Press Incline (p. 64)
One-Leg Chest Fly
   Incline (p. 84)

CORE
Knee Fold-Ups (p. 40)
Kneeling Layouts (p. 53)
Arm-Swing Rolls (p. 65)
Jackknifes (p. 85)

LEGS (THIGHS)
Hamstring Curls (p. 42)
Drop Squats (p. 54)
Thigh Buster (p. 66)
Scissors Lift (p. 86)

LEGS (BUTT/CALVES)
Butt Lift (p. 44)
Calf Raises (p. 55)
Atlas Lunge (p. 68)
One-Leg Drop Squat (p. 88)

SHOULDERS
Push-Offs (p. 45)
Right-Angle Lateral
   Lifts (p. 56)
Flying Carpet (p. 69)
Lateral Lifts (p. 89)

TRICEPS
Triceps Ball Press (p. 46)
Bridge Triceps Press (p. 58)
Triceps Extension (p. 70)
One-Legged Triceps Ball
   Press (p. 90)

Work Opposing Muscles   An example of opposing muscles is the biceps along the front of your arms and the triceps along the back. When your biceps contract, your triceps stretch. When your triceps contract, your biceps stretch. Other opposing muscle groups include your chest and upper back, your abs and lower back, and your quadriceps and hamstrings. Pairing exercises like this allows you to move through your workout faster because you won't need to rest in between. As you work your biceps, for instance, your triceps are already resting.

Add More Reps and More Weight   If you started with a light ball and you can easily do 15 repetitions, try a heavier ball.

For maximum results, you want to achieve "muscle failure" by the end of each exercise. In other words, you want to feel as if you couldn't perform one more repetition. On some exercises, you may need to perform as many as 20 or 30 repetitions to achieve failure. This helps build the kind of muscle endurance you use every day to carry heavy packages and do other tasks. Performing a high number of repetitions with a lower weight builds a sleeker muscle than doing fewer repetitions with a heavier weight.

Change Your Body Position   You can increase the challenge of any exercise by bringing more of your body off the ball. If you're doing the push-up from chapter 2, for example, balance with only the tops of your feet or toes on the fitness ball (see photo A). This also works for

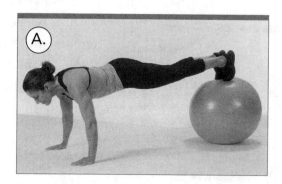

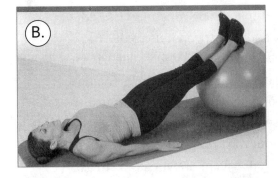

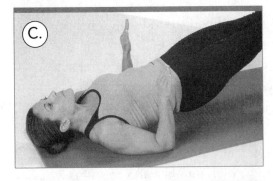

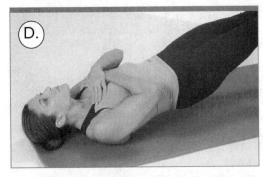

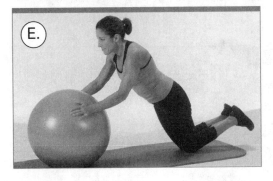

exercises such as the Butt Lift and Hamstring Curls (see photo B).

For exercises such as the Butt Lift where you are in reverse bridge, you can bring your hands in closer to your body to make the exercise more difficult. You can also try raising your forearms off the floor (see photo C). The toughest hand position of all is to cross your hands over your chest (see photo D). When your hands are crossed, you can't use them for balance and therefore must completely balance with your feet on the ball.

For exercises that require you to use your hands to press on the ball—such as Kneeling Layouts on page 53—you can increase the difficulty by placing only your forearms on the ball (see photo E).

Push the Speed   Increasing the intensity of your ball workout will not only burn more calories but also boost your fitness level. As you adapt to the exercises, you'll find you won't need to rest as much. When this happens, try moving fluidly from one exercise directly into the next with no rest time.

Ten New Moves

The ten exercises on the pages that follow are the toughest of the tough because they require you to balance by lifting a foot off the floor or by putting less of your body on the fitness ball. Some of these exercises also combine two motions to challenge your coordination.

Abs

OBLIQUE TWIST

The Oblique Twist starts like the Classic Crunch from chapter 2. By adding a twist, however, you work your obliques, or the muscles along the sides of your abdomen. The twisting action also requires you to work harder to stay balanced on the ball.

(A.) Sit on the fitness ball with your knees bent and your feet flat on the floor. Lean back and walk your body down the ball until the ball presses into your lower back. Place your fingers behind your head with your thumbs along your jawbone. Place your elbows out to the sides. Keep your back straight.

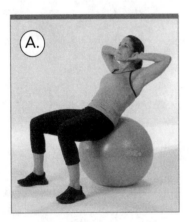 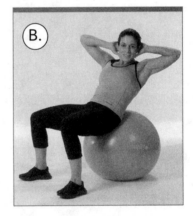

(B.) Exhale as you lift and twist your torso to the left, bringing your right shoulder toward your left hip. Inhale and return to center. Exhale and twist to the right. Repeat 4 to 5 times to each side.

Ball Basics

- Keep your elbows out to the sides as you twist. If you can see your elbows, you may be using your arms to pull your torso into the twist, and this can hurt your neck.

- The more of your torso that's off the ball, the more challenging the exercise. To increase the challenge, start the move with only your buttocks against the ball.

- For more challenge, extend your arms overhead.

- For even more challenge, move your feet closer together.

Back (Upper)

ALTERNATING FLIES

Alternating Flies is a variation on the Stomach Back Flies you learned in chapter 2. By lifting only one arm at a time, you are adding a balancing challenge. In Stomach Back Flies, you placed your feet farther apart—pointing toward 8 and 4 o'clock. In this exercise, bring your feet closer together to create less stability.

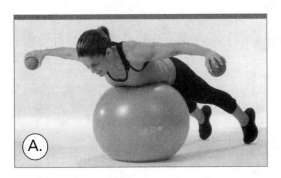

A. Lie in a prone position with your tummy on the ball, your legs extended, and your toes on the floor. Point your left leg toward 7 o'clock and your right toward 5 o' clock. Grasp a heavy ball in each hand. Extend your arms to your sides and raise them, bringing your shoulder blades closer together.

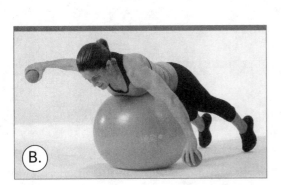

B. Inhale and lower your left hand toward the floor (but don't allow the ball to touch the floor). As you do so, keep your right arm extended and parallel to the floor. Exhale and raise your left arm back to the starting position. Then inhale and lower your right. Continue to alternate right and left for 10 to 15 complete repetitions on each side.

Ball Basics

- Try not to rest during this exercise. Keep both heavy balls off the floor at all times.

- For an even greater challenge, bring your feet closer together.

Back (Lower)

TORSO LIFT AND TWIST

Adding a twist to the Upper Torso Lift you learned in chapter 2 takes quite a bit of balance and coordination. The twisting action tones your back, buttocks, thighs, and sides.

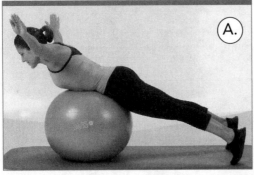

A. Place the ball in the middle of the mat. Lie in a prone position with your tummy on the ball. Place the balls of your feet on the floor, with your right leg pointing toward 5 o'clock and your left toward 7 o'clock. Extend your arms overhead.

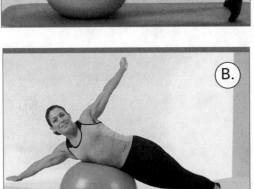

B. Exhale as you lift and twist your torso to the left, keeping your hips stationary. Inhale and return to center. Repeat to the right. Continue to alternate sides 10 to 15 times.

Ball Basics

- You can make the Torso Lift and Twist even more challenging by holding a pair of heavy balls with your arms extended from your sides at 90-degree angles to your torso.

- To increase the challenge of this exercise, bring your feet closer together.

Biceps

OFF-THE-BALL CURLS

Yes, this exercise looks much like the Off-the-Ball Curls you did in chapter 2. But notice my right leg. It's not on the floor! Anytime you want to make any exercise tougher, lift one foot off the floor.

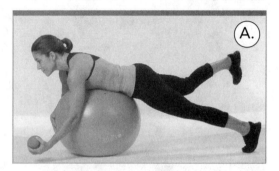

(A.) Lie with your tummy on the ball and your legs extended behind you, with the balls of your feet on the floor. Shift your body to the left so that only the right edge of your torso remains on the ball. Hug the ball with your right arm. Grasp a heavy ball in your left hand. Lift your right leg off the floor. Lift the heavy ball off the floor.

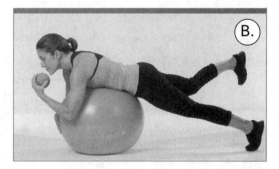

(B.) Exhale as you curl your left hand toward your left shoulder. Inhale and lower. Repeat 10 to 15 times and then switch sides.

Ball Basics

• When you lower the heavy ball, don't allow it to touch the floor.

• To increase the challenge even more, try lifting the leg on the same side as the arm that you are curling.

Chest

ONE-LEGGED CHEST FLY INCLINE

The One-Legged Chest Fly Incline looks somewhat like the Chest Fly you learned in chapter 2, but with two main differences: Extending

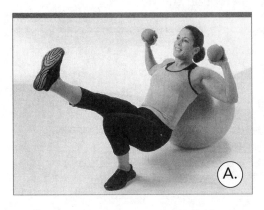

one leg makes it much harder to balance. Also, doing the move in an incline position, rather than in a full bridge, slightly changes the area of the chest that you tone, helping create the illusion of cleavage.

A. Sit on the fitness ball and slowly walk your body down the ball until it rests against your upper back. Keep your knees bent, your feet flat on the floor, and your buttocks a few inches below your knees. Grasp a heavy ball in each hand, and bring your elbows out to your sides at shoulder level. Your elbows should be bent, and your palms should be facing forward. Lift your right foot off the floor.

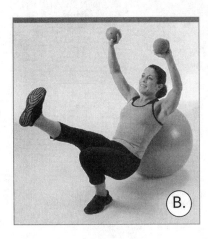

B. Exhale as you press the heavy balls toward one another in a large arcing motion, bringing your chest muscles toward one another. Inhale and lower. Repeat 10 to 15 times.

Ball Basics

- Keep your abs and buttocks tight throughout the exercise.

- To make this move harder, slide farther away from the ball, so that only your shoulders rest against it.

Core

JACKKNIFES

Remember the Knee Fold-Ups from chapter 2? Jackknifes require you to perform a similar motion, but this time your legs will be extended.

A. Get in the push-up position with the balls of your feet on the ball and your palms on the floor under your collarbones. Your body should form a straight line from your heels to your head.

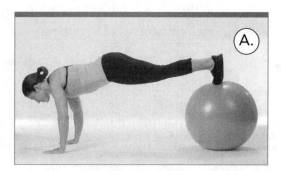

B. Exhale as you use your feet to pull the ball toward your hands. Keep your legs extended and raise your buttocks until they are directly above your hands (this requires concentration). Inhale and lower. Repeat up to 10 times.

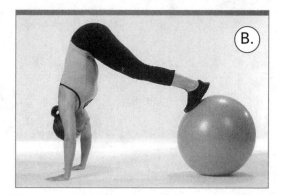

Ball Basics

- Keep your entire core tight throughout this move.

Legs (Thighs)

SCISSORS LIFT

Hugging the ball between your legs as you lift them takes some coordination. Once you master this exercise, however, you'll be able to simultaneously target your inner and outer thighs, buttocks, sides, and core muscles—all in one move.

(A.) Lie on your back with the ball between your legs. Roll onto your left side and prop up your head with your left palm above your ear. Rest your right hand on the mat in front of your tummy, similar to a bike's kickstand. Angle your right hip forward so that your right leg is about 6 inches in front of your left. Your legs will look like open scissors.

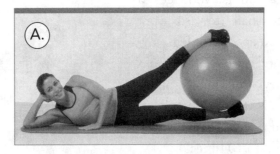

(B.) Exhale as you lift the ball directly toward the ceiling. Inhale and lower. Repeat 10 to 15 times. You will feel the movement in your inner and outer thighs, buttocks, and abs. Roll onto your back and then onto your right side and repeat.

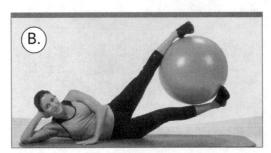

Ball Basics

- Use the strength of your abs to keep your torso motionless throughout this exercise.

- To increase the difficulty even more, try putting both hands behind your head.

Legs (Butt/Calves)

ONE-LEG DROP SQUAT

This exercise is just like the Drop Squat you learned in chapter 2, except now you only use one foot for balance. Not only is this move great for your rear but it also works your abs.

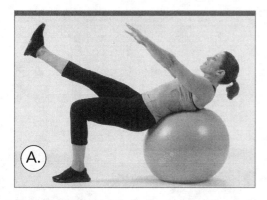

A. Lie in a bridge position with your upper back against the ball, your knees bent, and your feet flat on the floor. Extend your arms in front of you at chest level. Lift your right foot off the floor, extending it straight out from your hips.

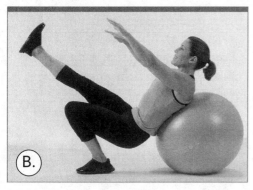

B. Inhale and squat down as you bend your left knee and sink your buttocks toward the floor. Allow the ball to roll as your back moves downward. Exhale and press back up through your left foot. Repeat 10 to 15 times, then switch legs.

Ball Basics

• To make the move even harder, cross your arms over your chest.

Shoulders

LATERAL LIFTS

In the Lateral Lift, you elevate one foot off the floor, making your abs, thighs, and back work hard to keep you balanced.

(A.) Sit on the fitness ball. Grasp a heavy ball in each hand. Lift your right foot off the floor and extend your leg.

(B.) As you keep your leg extended, exhale and lift your arms up laterally out to your sides, then raise them to shoulder height. Inhale and lower. Repeat 5 times. Keep your arms extended at shoulder height, switch legs, and repeat 5 times.

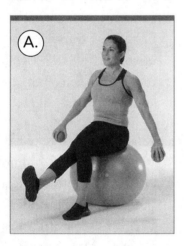 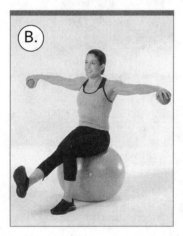

Ball Basics

- For variety, you can do alternating lateral lifts. Lift one arm in front and the other to the side, then switch sides.

Triceps

ONE-LEGGED TRICEPS BALL PRESS

I saved the hardest move for last. The Triceps Ball Press in chapter 2 requires you to maintain quite a bit of balance. Now you'll do the move with only one leg on the ball. This is also a great workout for your buttocks and the backs of your thighs.

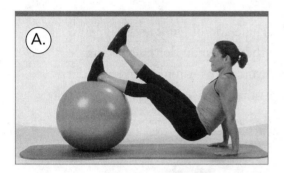

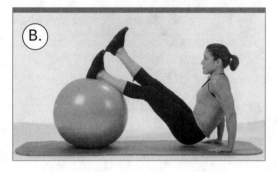

A. Sit on the mat with your hands behind your buttocks on either side of your hips. Place your left calf on top of the ball and elevate your right calf a couple inches above the ball. Press through the palms of your hands to lift your buttocks off the mat as you straighten your elbows.

B. Inhale and bend your elbows to lower your torso, but don't allow your buttocks to touch the floor. Exhale and press back to the starting position. Repeat 10 to 15 times.

Ball Basics

- Don't rest between repetitions. Keep your buttocks off the mat at all times.

PART TWO

the six-week
body makover

4

your six-week body makeover

The elements of success

I have yet to meet a woman who *didn't* want to make over her body. Every day, it seems, my female students, colleagues, friends, workout partners, and acquaintances all ask me the following questions:

- "How can I shrink my hips, thighs, and butt?"

- "I liked my body until I started menopause. Now, despite following my fitness program, I'm gaining weight in my belly. How do I stop it?"

- "My metabolism won't budge. I eat less and less, but I still can't lose weight."

- "No matter how many leg lifts I do, my thighs never get smaller. What am I doing wrong?"

Part of these weight "problems" is actually in our heads. To us women, the slightest bulge seems extremely noticeable, if only to us! The other part of the problem is physical, and it results from our unique genetics. Women gain weight more easily than do men, and we have a tougher time losing it. Female fat cells are stubborn, and you need a combination approach to control them. Therefore, you want a body makeover program that includes the following:

- Strength training
- Cardiovascular exercise
- Smart eating
- Motivational cues

I'll explain each of those concepts soon, but first, let's take a look at female fat and why it sticks with and to us.

The Frustrating Nature of the Female Fat Cell

Women have more body fat than do men, and the reason is simple: We need fuel in the form of fat to support us during pregnancy and to produce milk when we breast-feed our infants.

Also, because our genetics haven't changed in thousands of years, we still possess the physiology of our cave-dwelling ancestors. Back then, the woman who had the ability to store plenty of fat was able to survive the harsh conditions, live into adulthood, and have children. These cave women often carried extra fat in their hips and thighs that served as fuel for pregnancy and lactation when food was scarce. Ultimately, the offspring of these cave women passed on their genetics to succeeding generations and down to us.

If you're of childbearing age and have the body shape of a pear, you can thank your cave women ancestors. They passed on an enzyme called lipoprotein lipase (LPL), which makes fat in the hip, thigh, and buttock region particularly hard to lose. LPL sits on the surface of all fat cells and is responsible for filling the cell with energy reserves. LPL is more active in the hip-thigh region in women than elsewhere in the body, which explains why this site is a fat depot for many of us.

Your Body, Your Self

I'm all for doing the most with what you have, and I'm excited that you've chosen to tackle this body makeover.

That said, if I could have one wish for every woman, it would be that she learn to love her unique shape and not want to look like someone else. Your body shape is yours, a blend of your genetics and femaleness. The body shape you see on others and may desire for yourself may not be possible with your particular genetics.

Women who have a "perfect" shape usually have fewer fat cells in their hips and thighs and therefore less storage area. They have the ideal scenario for smaller legs, thighs, and hips. Don't compare yourself with those women. As you go along your body makeover journey, focus on your best efforts to improve yourself, not on how your body compares with other women.

Another enzyme called hormone sensitive lipase (HSL) helps our fat cells release their fat when the body needs fuel.

In other parts of our body, the process of storing and releasing fat usually runs smoothly, like saving money in a bank account and then accessing it later with an ATM card. Fat disbursement from the hips and thighs, however, is different. This fat is like money tied up in a long-term investment that isn't readily accessible. These fat cells like to store and hold onto fat rather than relinquish it. This is why, when we diet, we tend to lose fat from elsewhere in the body but not from the thigh region.

When we enter menopause, we experience the lowering of our sex hormone levels. As this happens, our fat cells get the message that they no longer need to hold onto hip and thigh fat for childbearing. So, now fat starts bulging in the abdominal area, and we take on the shape

Six Weeks to a New You

Remember this important fact: Weight loss takes time.

By the time many women decide they want to lose weight, they're completely disgusted with their looks and want the extra pounds off *yesterday*. They don't take into account that putting on those extra pounds took a few years, and taking them off will also take time. Although your weight loss during the exercise ball program won't take years, you should allow yourself about one week for every 1 to 2 pounds you want to lose.

This program lasts six weeks because that's how much time it takes for most women to see noticeable results. If you have many pounds to lose, you may need to wait as many as fifteen weeks or more before you hit your final weight-loss goal.

Remember, your true goal isn't sticking to the program for six or twelve or eighteen or more weeks. You want to stick with it for the rest of your life. That's the only way to stay off the dieting roller coaster once and for all.

of a man. This type of fat is particularly dangerous, because it is linked to heart disease. As muscle mass shrinks, our metabolism slows, and not surprisingly, we gain weight more easily.

All women posses a propensity toward a pear shape before menopause and an apple shape afterward. Our individual genetics determine why this happens more dramatically in some women than in others. The good news: You can fight back against your genetics—at any age. Your fight will require the four-pronged approach I mentioned earlier: strength training, cardiovascular exercise, smart eating, and motivational cues. Let's take a look at each of these weapons in the battle against female fat.

Strength Training

As you learned in chapter 1, strength training builds muscle and boosts your metabolism by as much as 100 more burned calories a day. Muscle also adds shape to your body, giving your legs a sleek curve, lifting your buttocks, and adding definition to your arms and shoulders. In your abdomen, muscle acts like a girdle and holds your internal organs in place.

Many women fail to see results from strength training, however, because they target only the parts of their bodies that they want to shrink. Such "spot-reducing" workouts aren't effective because you need muscle all over your body to boost your metabolism, not just in your butt or thighs. In fact, doing toning moves only in the legs may do exactly the opposite of what you want. Your legs may appear larger as fat stores fail to shrink and the muscles begin to grow.

Believe it or not, to truly change your body shape, you must build up your shoulders. The reason? Good shoulders create the illusion of smaller hips.

Also, you must build enough calorie-hungry muscle throughout your body to increase your metabolism. In short, the best strength-training program for weight loss and spot reducing is a total body strength-training program. The fitness ball provides faster results and a more efficient workout than just about anything else, because you work multiple muscles at once.

The strength-training routines outlined in this six-week makeover mix and match the exercises in chapter 2. Every two weeks of the program you take on a new set of exercises from that chapter. Each routine will seem slightly different from the one you did the day before. In some cases I've simply rearranged the order of exercises, allowing you to work your muscles in a different order from your last workout. In others, I've included an entirely new set of exercises.

This constant variety will help keep you mentally entertained and will help you stick with your program. It will also work your muscles in new ways and make your workouts more effective. Consistently changing the types of exercises you do will fully work different areas of individual muscles and give them a sleek shape. Your muscles will also work harder, because you're much less likely to cheat when an exercise feels foreign to you.

You'll find the suggested workouts in the six-week workbook provided in chapter 7.

Cardiovascular Exercise

You probably know that cardiovascular exercise, such as walking, helps burn calories. For every mile you walk or run, you burn roughly 100 calories.

Cardiovascular exercise helps make over your body in another important way as well. It helps trick your fat cells into releasing their cargo. Think again about our cave-dwelling ancestors. Their bodies began to hold onto fat when food was scarce, when cave-dwelling Jane moved little to gather food (because there was no food to gather). This is why our modern bodies respond to our physical movements as cues to hold onto fat or to release it. When you exercise aerobically, your body gets the message that food is plentiful. It stops running so efficiently and allows your body to burn more fat. This encourages your fat cells to let go of their cargo, assuming you don't counter your efforts by overeating.

In chapters 6 and 7, you'll learn how to incorporate cardiovascular exercise into your makeover program for maximum results.

Smart Eating

Your exercise habits will only help you shed fat if you are smart about eating and if you don't eat extra food to replace the calories you burn during your exercise sessions.

You also don't want to sabotage your weight-loss campaign by cutting *too many* calories from your diet. Studies show that drastic dieting or calorie cutting makes LPL activity climb. As we have seen, this causes the body to conserve energy and hold on tightly to stored fat. You need modest calorie cutting of only 100 to 500 calories per day to coax fat out of storage, calorie by calorie.

Some lucky women may actually need to eat *more* to lose weight. Our bodies actually burn calories just by digesting and processing food. Smaller, more frequent meals help bolster metabolism, particularly in women who may have undermined their metabolism in the past with frequent crash diets.

Another dieting pitfall occurs when we cut back on fatty foods and fill ourselves up instead with fat-free foods that are rich in carbohydrates. Fat-free cookies and crackers only make us feel deprived of fat, yet they contain almost the same number of calories.

In chapter 5, you'll find my dessert diet, a food plan designed to allow maximum food enjoyment by including dessert every single day. The plan helps you pinpoint your true calorie needs. Once you know how many calories you can have each day, you pick an easy-to-follow weight-loss pyramid that helps you automatically eat the right foods in the right amounts every day without feeling deprived.

Motivational Cues

If weight loss were as easy as watching what we eat and adding more exercise to the mix, we'd all look like supermodels.

The truth is, we all have days when we just don't feel like sticking with our weight-loss program. By designing fun workouts and a no-deprivation eating plan, I hope to have provided you with a program that you will want to follow every day. However, to help you surmount occasional boredom and, yes, laziness, I've also included some motivational help.

The six-week workbook in chapter 7 includes numerous checklists, tips, and reflective questions for you to read, think about, and even write about during every single day of the program. These check-lists and questions will keep you honest. Research shows that the simple act of writing down the food we eat every day can serve as a powerful motivational force in making better food choices.

Not only will the tips help increase your willpower, but they will also actually make willpower less necessary. Every day of the program you'll find a new tip to help you eat better, feel better, and lose weight. These tips make smart eating and exercise fun and automatic. Many of them come from my personal life. They are the very things I do to stay fit and firm into my forties.

5

why every dieter
needs dessert

And why reduced fat and nonfat foods
just don't cut the mustard

I believe in chocolate. I believe in premium ice cream. I believe in self-indulgence.

The floor of my car is often littered with chocolate candy wrappers. My favorite restaurant is the local Ben and Jerry's ice cream shop. My family knows where I keep my chocolate stash—and they know to keep their hands off.

Despite all this naughtiness, however, I've been able to maintain my weight at a trim 120 pounds for the past twenty-some years. I'm happy to tell you that you can experience the same results—and eat chocolate or ice cream or some other decadent dessert every single day.

Skeptical? Are you wondering if I'm one of those genetic anomalies, one of those fortunate people with a fast metabolism? Are you wondering if this is just another diet gimmick, like the cabbage soup diet or the food-combining diet?

If you are, the answer to both questions is no.

Before we look at why my dessert diet works, let's first see why diets that ban dessert *don't* work. During the past twenty years, an abundance of deprivation-centered weight-loss programs have claimed that eliminating one type of food or another from a woman's diet will help her lose weight. Perhaps you've tried one—or many—of these diets.

Perhaps you gave up chocolate or cookies or pie. Do you remember feeling fixated on food, restraining your eating, omitting entire food groups, and feeling *very* guilty if you cheated? Whenever you cut an entire food group out of your diet—and dessert *is* a food group—you crave it more than ever. It's one of the laws of life: We want what we can't have.

Diets that require us to cut out our favorite foods fail because they go against the very grain of our being. Most of us have enough willpower to forgo our favorite foods for a week or maybe even a month. Few of us possess the willpower to give them up forever. To lose weight and keep it off, you must make dietary changes that you can sustain for the rest of your life. Otherwise, you will return to your old eating habits, and the weight will return, usually with extra padding.

That's why I encourage you to go right ahead and eat your favorite foods. Eating means more than maintaining a balance of vitamins, minerals, and phytochemicals. It's also about comfort and joy. When you cut entire foods out of your life or force yourself to eat the not-so-tasty reduced fat and reduced-calorie versions exclusively, you lose the natural joy of eating.

The truth is, to lose weight, you need to cut calories—it doesn't matter where they come from. So why make them come from the foods you love the most? Why not take them from foods that don't call your name so loudly? Why make weight loss about willpower when you can make it an exercise in joyful eating?

Let's face it, dessert is comfort food. Scientists now know that the sugar and fat combination of many desserts helps boost levels of the soothing brain chemical serotonin. Research shows that low levels of this important chemical can bring on the anxiety or depression often associated with binge eating. Dosing yourself daily with a serotonin-boosting food will go a long way to helping you control your eating.

On my dessert diet, you will learn how to build a nutritious base to your diet and still savor your favorite foods. Yes, you'll eat a few foods that are "fattening" and that may offer little in the way of nutrition, but they will go a long way toward satisfying your soul. These foods will be offset by an abundance of other foods that supply a wealth of important health- and energy-promoting nutrients.

This isn't a diet gimmick. Each day you will consume optimal amounts of vitamins, minerals, and phytochemicals—without feeling deprived! I'll show you how to fill up on quality calories, while you enjoy the natural goodness of fruits, vegetables, healthful fats, and whole grains.

On the program, I'll also show you how you can regularly eat 200-calorie portions of your favorite desserts, while at the same time keeping your overall caloric intake low enough to lose weight. You will fall in love with eating all over again—and lose weight in the process!

Let's get started.

Get Acquainted with Calories

Your first step on the path to building a soul-satisfying dessert diet takes some detective work.

Before you can cut calories from your diet, you must first know how many calories you're eating on a regular basis compared with how many you *should* be eating. To lose a pound of fat, you need to eat 3,500 fewer calories than you burn. You will want to lose this weight slowly. Research shows that losing any more than 2 pounds a week can cause the body to go into starvation mode as the metabolism slows down to conserve calories.

To lose 1/2 to 2 pounds a week, you want to consume about 500 to 1,000 fewer calories per day than you are currently eating. (Your new fitness ball exercise program will burn an additional 250 to 500 calories a day, enough for slow but steady weight loss. To lose weight a little faster, you will combine the ball exercises with calorie cutting.)

To find out how many calories you generally eat and burn in a day, follow these steps.

Step 1   Get a handle on what you eat. Using the space provided in Your Food Diary on page 105, jot down exactly what *and* how much you eat in one day. Try to pick a day that represents your typical diet—try not to cheat by eating less on this day. Record everything you eat or drink. Include snacks, beverages, meals, condiments, and all those extra nibbles and bites that work their way into your tummy. Use a measuring cup for accuracy. Be sure also to use the chart How to Eyeball Portions on page 106 for visual comparisons. You don't want to fool yourself that you are eating a one-half cup of pasta when you're really eating a full cup with twice the calories!

After writing down all the foods you eat, tally your calorie total for the day. To get calorie counts of food, refer to the "Nutrition Facts" labels on packages and jars, a calorie-count book (available at most grocery store check-out magazine racks), or an online calorie counter like the one at www.dietwatch.com (see the link for "nutrition calculator").

Write your daily calorie intake here: _____

Step 2   Pinpoint how many calories you actually *need*. Many women go wrong right here. In an effort to lose weight fast, they underestimate their food needs and cut too many calories from their diet. They end up slowing their metabolism and sabotaging their efforts.

Your body requires a minimum number of calories daily to fuel basic functions such as breathing, heart pumping, and brain activity. It needs an additional number to fuel muscles as they perform movements such as walking, sitting at a desk, waiting tables, and, of course, working out. Use this formula to compute the number of calories you should eat daily if you want to drop about 1/2 to 2 pounds per week:

11 calories × number of pounds of body weight = _____,
number of calories you need per day for weight loss

Your Food Diary

TIME	FOOD	PORTION SIZE	HOW PREPARED	CONDIMENTS	OTHER

For example, if you weigh 150 pounds and want to lose about 15 pounds over two to three months time, your formula would look like:

11 calories/pound × 150 pounds = 1650 calories daily

Write the number of calories you need for weight loss: _____

Step 3   Take your calorie intake from Step 1 and subtract from it the number of calories you need for weight loss from Step 2. This difference often shocks some of my clients. If you are overeating by only 100 calories a day, you will gain a pound of extra weight in just five weeks!

Write the number of extra calories you're eating here: _____

Step 4   Now it's time to pick your dessert diet food pyramid from pages 119 to 121. Keep in mind that you never want to cut more than

How to Eyeball Portions

To make sure you have the right portion of food, use the following everyday comparisons.

1/2 cup pasta, cooked rice, mashed potatoes	=	chubby computer mouse
3 ounces cooked meat, fish, poultry	=	1 deck of playing cards
1 ounce cheese	=	2 cubes of dice
1 medium size piece of fruit	=	1 tennis ball
1 teaspoon margarine	=	top joint of thumb

500 calories at one time from your diet. Otherwise, you'll feel deprived and hungry and risk slowing your metabolism.

To choose your pyramid, do the following:

- First, look at your answer from Step 3. If it amounts to 500 or more calories, you'll choose your pyramid by subtracting 500 from your daily calorie intake from Step 1.

- If the difference is from 0 to 500 calories, choose the pyramid closest to your answer in Step 2. In other words, if your Step 2 answer equals 1450 calories, you'll use the 1500-calorie pyramid.

- Use a green pen and draw a star or checkmark next to the right pyramid for you. Keep in mind that your pyramid may change as you lose weight. For every 5 pounds you lose, go through Step 1 through Step 3 again, just to make sure you are following the correct pyramid.

- When you achieve your weight-loss goal and want to maintain your weight and not lose any more, use this formula:

14 calories × number of pounds of body weight = _____, number of calories you need to maintain weight

Choose Your Dessert

Now it's time to have some fun and choose your dessert. Please, don't feel tempted to rush along your weight loss by skipping this important step. Eating dessert every day provides the foundation for this eating plan. If you skip this step, you will have an eating plan with a very shaky foundation.

Every woman can fit 150 to 200 calories a day worth of soul-satisfying food into her diet. Yes, even you. Yes, even if you are already overeating on a regular basis.

You'll soon learn how to lower your daily calorie total by making smarter food choices. Right now, however, you are going to take steps to ensure you will lose weight without feeling deprived.

Everyone has self-indulgent foods that they hate to give up. My self-indulgent foods include chocolate, especially when dipped in peanut butter, and ice cream. Perhaps your self-indulgent foods include apple pie. Or maybe you feel self-indulgent when you eat a non-dessertlike beef jerky or bread dipped in olive oil. To count a food as self-indulgent, you have to feel guilty, as if you've cheated on your diet, when you eat it.

Maybe you try to limit these foods by not stocking them in your pantry. Nevertheless, at some point they get the better of you, and you suddenly find yourself eating not one but two or three chocolate bars.

Here's how to get in control of these foods and not allow them to control you.

1. Identify your top five to seven most self-indulgent foods. Write them in the space provided.

_____

_____

_____

_____

_____

_____

_____

2. Schedule these foods into your diet. With careful planning, you can fit 150 to 200 calories of dessert and other types of "junk food" into your diet. Once you realize that controlled small portions of your favorite foods aren't going to make you fat or ruin your health, your self-

indulgent foods will lose their power over you. Each day, allow yourself to savor a self-indulgent food—you won't binge because you'll know that you only have to wait until tomorrow to have some more.

Next to each food on your self-indulgent food list, write down how much and how often you plan to eat it. To help you arrive at the right serving sizes of your favorite foods, I've listed more than fifty common desserts and self-indulgent foods, along with a suggested serving size.

DESSERT/INDULGENT FOODS	QUANTITY	CALORIES
After Eight Mints	8 mints	120
Animal crackers	12 pieces	140
Beef jerky	2 large pieces	165
Bit-O-Honey bar	1.7 ounces	190
Boston cream pie (frozen)	1/8 of a cake	180
Brownie (2-inch square)	1	140
Butterscotch chips	2 tablespoons	160
Candy corn	1/4 cup	180
Caramels	5 pieces	170
Carrot cake (homemade)	1/24 of a 9-inch cake	200
Cheesecake	1/24 of a 9-inch cake	200
Cheese puffs	1 ounce	150
Chips Ahoy chocolate chip cookies	3 cookies	160
Chocolate cake	1/12 of a 9-inch cake	200
Chocolate-covered almonds	1 ounce (8 almonds)	160
Chocolate-covered peanuts	9 peanuts	200
Chocolate-covered raisins	1.6 ounces	190
Chocolate fudge sandwich cookie	2 cookies	165
Coffee cake with crumb topping	1/12 of an 8-inch cake	200
Corn chips	1 ounce	155
Cupcake with icing	1 cupcake	170
Dark chocolate	1.3 ounces	200

(continues)

DESSERT/INDULGENT FOODS	QUANTITY	CALORIES
Doughnut, cake	1 doughnut	200
Fudge	1.2 ounces	130
Gum drops	10 small pieces	135
Gummy bears	1.4 ounces	130
Hot fudge topping	2 tablespoons	140
Ice cream, coffee (Haagen-Dazs)	1/3 cup	170
Ice cream, vanilla (16% fat)	1/2 cup	180
Jelly beans	15 large	150
Jelly crème pie, Little Debbie	1 pie	156
M & Ms	55 pieces	190
M & Ms peanut	20 pieces	200
Marshmallows	8 large	195
Milk chocolate	1 ounce	155
Milky Way bar	3/4 of 2.15-ounce bar	195
Nestlé Crunch bar	1.4 ounces	200
Oatmeal cookies (2 1/2 inches)	2 cookies	160
Oreos	2 cookies	160
Peanut brittle	1 ounce	130
Peanut butter cookie (2 1/4 inches)	2	160
Peanut butter cup (Reese's)	1	135
Pie, apple	1/10 of a 9-inch pie	200
Pie, chocolate cream	1/16 of a 9-inch pie	200
Potato chips	1 ounce	152
Pound cake	1 ounce	130
Semi-sweet chocolate chips	2 tablespoons	160
Shortbread (Lorna Doone)	4 cookies	140
Snickers bar	2/3 of a 2.16-ounce bar	200
Taffy	1.5 ounces (3 pieces)	175
Toffee	1 ounce	160
Tortilla chips, nacho flavor	1 ounce	156
Truffle	1-ounce piece	140

Smarten Up Your Diet

Now that you've picked your favorite dessert, you're ready to cut calories from other foods. Eating the *right* foods supplies your body with the necessary ingredients for your weight-loss metamorphosis. You will need to eat vital proteins, essential fats, energizing carbohydrates, and rejuvenating fluids along with enriching vitamins and minerals.

Some diet experts like to split foods into two categories: bad foods and good foods. I don't like to do that, because it stirs up those dangerous guilty feelings. We all recognize that some foods are better for us than others. I like to think of some foods as "troublesome" foods, meaning foods that we crave, that are high in calories, and that don't contain the nutrients for weight loss. I think of other foods as "smart" foods, those that are naturally lower in calories and packed with nutrition.

Here's how to make smarter food choices.

Eat Smart Protein Foods   Smart protein sources are low in fat and high in all the building blocks—zinc, iron, copper, and B vitamins—needed for rebuilding and strengthening muscle and cartilage, as well as bolstering a healthy immune system. Smart protein foods also take time to digest and help us feel full for a longer period of time, thus avoiding the "hungries" that can sometimes lead to overeating.

There are also troublesome protein foods that add extra fat to our diets and contain little in the way of extra nutrition. See Make the Smart Switch: Proteins for a list of smart and troublesome protein choices.

Take a look at the protein sources—the meats, dairy products, beans, fish, and soy foods that you listed in Step 1 of Get Acquainted with Calories. Circle your troublesome protein foods with a red marker. Circle your smart protein sources with a green marker. Use the space that follows to write down a few different smart protein foods that you plan to eat for meals and snacks. These might include yogurt topped with fruit for breakfast, a chicken burrito for lunch, soy nuts with raisins

Make the Smart Switch: Proteins

SMART PROTEIN CHOICES

Tofu

Veggie burgers

Veggie dogs

Veggie cheese

Veggie ground round

Veggie lunchmeat

Soy milk

Fish

Shellfish

Top round beef

Beef sirloin

Chicken without the skin

Nonfat or lowfat dairy yogurt
   or milk

Turkey without the skin

Ground turkey without the skin

Pork loin

Extra lean ground beef (less
   than 8% fat)

Ham, lean

Lean deli meats (roast beef,
   turkey)

TROUBLESOME PROTEIN CHOICES

Prime rib

Ground beef

Beef franks

Full-fat dairy (whole milk,
   yogurt)

Cheese (Swiss, cheddar,
   Monterey jack)

Fried fish

Fried meat

Sausages

Ham, fatty

High-fat deli meats (pastrami,
   salami)

Lamb

for a snack, and grilled fish over rice for dinner. Every day, try to make at least one smarter protein choice than you did the day before.

_____

_____

_____

_____

Make the Smart Switch: Fats

SMART FAT CHOICES

Peanut butter and other nut
   butters

Nuts (almond, walnuts,
   pecans, macadamias)

Olive oil

Avocado and guacamole
   (without added fat)

Trans-free margarine

Reduced fat margarine

Low or nonfat dairy products

Low or nonfat cheese

Vegetable-oil-based salad
   dressings

TROUBLESOME FAT CHOICES

Butter

Margarine (hard stick)

Non-oil-based salad dressings

Full-fat diary products (cream,
   half and half, sour cream)

Mayonnaise

Croissants and other high-fat
   bakery items

Eat Smart Fats   Smart fats include monounsaturated and omega-3 fatty acids. These two types of fat rejuvenate the skin, sustain a healthy immune system, and help ward off ailments such as cancer and heart disease. Foods that contain these fats include nuts, nut oils, fish and other seafood, and flaxseed oil or meal.

Troublesome fats include foods composed of saturated fat found in animal products and trans fats found in fried and processed foods that list "hydrogenated" and "partially hydrogenated" oils on the ingredients list. These include margarine, cream cheese, fatty meats, fried foods, some oils, and salad dressings. Troublesome fats occur in cookies, crackers, baked goods, and fast foods. Many of these foods supply nothing more than saturated and trans fat calories and contain virtually zero in the essential fat department. Look for trans-fat free margarine and other foods.

Go to your food diary and circle the "troublesome fats" with a red marker and the "smart fats" with a green marker. Then, in the space provided, write smart fat substitutes for the troublesome fats that you circled. See Make the Smart Switch: Fats for a list of troublesome and smart fats. Every day, try to make at least one smarter fat choice than you did the day before.

_____

_____

_____

_____

_____

_____

Eat Smart Carbohydrates   Smart carbohydrate foods provide a wealth of energizing fuel, fiber, vitamins, minerals, and health-boosting phytochemicals such as flavonoids. They include oatmeal and other fiber-rich breakfast cereals, whole grain breads and pastas, baked quinoa and bulgur, and all fruits and vegetables.

Troublesome carbohydrate foods include plain pasta and white bread and other foods made from refined white flour. They also may be loaded with sugar, as in candy and cookies. While these foods pack a good dose of carbohydrates that your muscles and brain use for fuel, there's little else here in the way of vitamins and minerals or fiber that your body needs for top performance and health. (However, if you listed any carbohydrate foods as your "self-indulgent foods," you'll be working them into your diet, not subtracting them out. Carbohydrates only become troublesome when you eat them mindlessly).

Now, go to your food diary and circle all of the troublesome carbohydrate foods with a red marker and the smart carbohydrate foods with a green marker. See Make the Smart Switch: Carbohydrates for a list of smart and troublesome carbohydrate choices.

Make the Smart Switch: Carbohydrates

SMART CARBOHYDRATE CHOICES

Fruit (all types, no sugar
   added if canned or frozen)
Vegetables (all types)
Breads, pasta, and cooked
   whole grains such as whole
   wheat, quinoa, barley, rye,
   and millet

Oatmeal
Nine-grain cereal
Whole grain ready-to-eat
   breakfast cereals
Brown rice

TROUBLESOME CARBOHYDRATE CHOICES

Chips
Crackers
White bread, bagels

Plain pasta
Bakery muffins

In the space provided, list smart carbohydrate choices that you can substitute for the troublesome carbohydrate foods you tend to eat. Every day, try to make at least one smarter carbohydrate choice than you did the day before.

_____

_____

_____

_____

_____

Drink Smart Fluids Smart fluids include plain old water—carbonated or not—as well as low-calorie, vitamin-rich beverages like tomato juice, low or noncalorie beverages such as sports drinks and diet drinks, and watery foods such as clear broth soups. (Though fresh fruits and vegetables contain a lot of water, they fall under "carbohydrate" foods.)

Smart fluids help energize the brain and body. Because our bodies contain a staggering 140-plus cups of water, daily replenishment is vital. We need water daily and lots of it. Fluids keep skin and brain cells plump with water, which of course has a direct impact on how we look and feel. Our muscles use water for cooling during a workout as well as a vehicle for nutrient delivery and waste disposal. Fluids also take up quite a bit of stomach volume, helping squelch feelings of hunger.

Troublesome fluids include those that contain lots of calories and no nutrition—such as soft drinks and most so-called fruit drinks—as well as those that contain caffeine, such as coffee and tea. Too much caffeine can leave you feeling jittery and zapped by the end of the day, not the feeling you want when it's time to do your ball workout.

Go to your food diary and circle your smart beverages with a green pen and your troublesome beverages in red. See Make the Smart Switch: Fluids for a list of troublesome and smart fluid choices.

You need to drink 2 cups of smart fluids for every 500 calories that you burn. Calculate this based on your answer in Step 2 of Get Acquainted with Calories. In the space provided, write the smart fluids you plan to drink to meet your fluid needs. Consider starting off your day with a fresh glass of water. Take along a filled water bottle to drink at work (fill it up periodically at the water cooler), and always bring water, fitness water, or a sports drink with you to the gym.

_____

_____

_____

_____

_____

Make the Smart Switch: Fluids

SMART FLUID CHOICES

Plain water

Carbonated water

Tea

Fitness water (very low calorie)

TROUBLESOME FLUID CHOICES

Soda (all types)

Fruit drinks

Sweetened teas

Energy drinks

Lemonade (commercial type)

Learn to Eyeball Calories

The final step of your dessert diet is portion control, and it may be the hardest.

Counting calories is time-consuming and tedious. Yet, to lose weight, you must stay under your caloric goal. That's why I've developed a food eyeballing system that helps you automatically figure out in your head the caloric wallop of every single meal—without having to search through a long list of foods.

Here's how to do it.

Choose the dessert diet pyramid (beginning on page 119) that most closely matches the caloric goal you chose in Get Acquainted with Calories.

Note the number of servings, serving size, and calorie count of each food group: grains, fruits, vegetables, meats and beans, dairy, and fats.

For the first few days, measure your foods using standard kitchen measuring cups to get a feel for what constitutes a serving. At the same time, use the chart on page 118, which shows common serving sizes of the foods you are eating. By doing these two things together,

What's a Serving?

Wholegrain breads/starches: 80 calories = 1 serving

1/2 bagel, 3 ounces baked potato, 1 slice bread, 3/4 cup cold cereal, 3 whole wheat crackers, 1/2 cup cooked pasta, 3 cups air-popped popcorn, 1/3 cup rice

Vegetables (1/2 cup cooked, 1 cup raw): 25 calories = 1 serving

broccoli, carrots, celery, green beans, snow peas, cabbage, green lettuce, onions, squash

Fruits (1 medium fruit of tennis ball size or 1/2 cup juice of any of the following): 60 calories = 1 serving

apple, apricot, banana, berries, grapes, kiwi fruit, peach, pear, melon, orange

Calcium-rich foods: 90–200 calories = 1 serving (check labels)

1 cup nonfat plain or fruit yogurt, 1 cup skim or 1 percent milk, 1 cup fortified soy milk

Protein-rich foods: Calories vary per serving (see below)

1 ounce fish (35 calories), 1 ounce poultry (50 calories), 1 ounce lean meat (60 calories), 1/4 cup nonfat, 1 percent cottage cheese (40 calories), 1 ounce part-skim, lowfat cheese (50–100 calories), 1 egg (70 calories), 1/2 cup tofu (100–150 calories), 1 tablespoon peanut butter, 1 cup cooked beans: lentils, kidney beans, etc. (180 calories = 1 meat and 2 servings starch)

Healthful fats/sweets: 35–45 calories = 1 serving

1 teaspoon margarine, 1 tablespoon diet margarine, 1 teaspoon regular mayonnaise, 1 tablespoon reduced-calorie mayonnaise, 1 teaspoon oil (olive, corn), 2 tablespoons reduced-calorie dressing, 1 1/2 tablespoon light cream cheese, 1 tablespoon chopped nuts, 1/2 ounce chocolate, 2 teaspoons honey

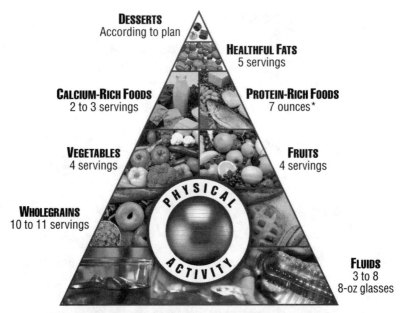

DESSERTS
According to plan

HEALTHFUL FATS
5 servings

CALCIUM-RICH FOODS
2 to 3 servings

PROTEIN-RICH FOODS
7 ounces*

VEGETABLES
4 servings

FRUITS
4 servings

WHOLEGRAINS
10 to 11 servings

PHYSICAL ACTIVITY

FLUIDS
3 to 8
8-oz glasses

Dessert-Diet Pyramid for 2000 Calories Per Day
*See list on page 118 for equivalents

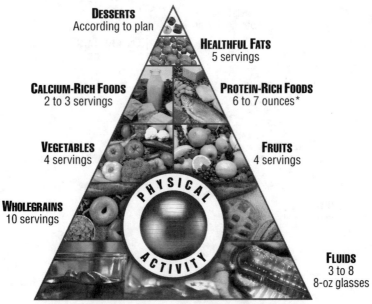

DESSERTS
According to plan

HEALTHFUL FATS
5 servings

CALCIUM-RICH FOODS
2 to 3 servings

PROTEIN-RICH FOODS
6 to 7 ounces*

VEGETABLES
4 servings

FRUITS
4 servings

WHOLEGRAINS
10 servings

PHYSICAL ACTIVITY

FLUIDS
3 to 8
8-oz glasses

Dessert-Diet Pyramid for 1800 Calories Per Day
*See list on page 118 for equivalents

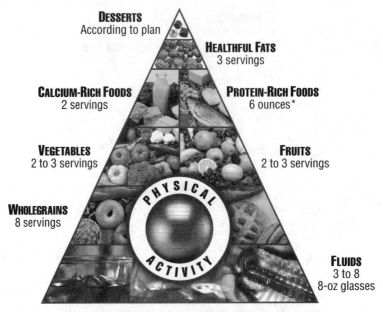

Dessert-Diet Pyramid for 1500 Calories Per Day
*See list on page 118 for equivalents

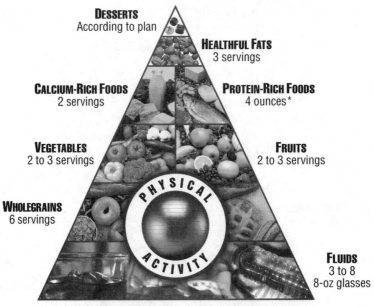

Dessert-Diet Pyramid for 1200 Calories Per Day
*See list on page 118 for equivalents

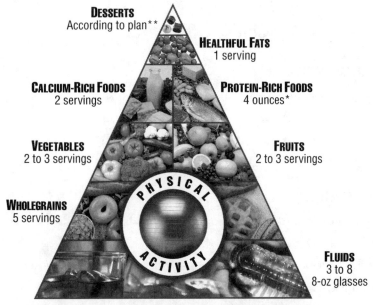

DESSERTS
According to plan**

HEALTHFUL FATS
1 serving

CALCIUM-RICH FOODS
2 servings

PROTEIN-RICH FOODS
4 ounces*

VEGETABLES
2 to 3 servings

FRUITS
2 to 3 servings

WHOLEGRAINS
5 servings

PHYSICAL ACTIVITY

FLUIDS
3 to 8
8-oz glasses

Dessert-Diet Pyramid for 1000 Calories Per Day
*See list on page 118 for equivalents
**Choose either a fat-free or lowfat dessert

you'll be able to eye any amount of food and immediately figure out how many servings there are.

To make your meals and snacks even easier to control, I've provided the Check-Off Charts on page 122 so you can check off servings of grains, fruits, vegetables, meats, beans, dairy, and fats as you eat them. There are different charts to correspond with different calorie goals. The number of boxes after each type of food indicates the number of servings you should eat each day. You can photocopy these charts and use them as long as you need. Once you've checked off all the boxes on your chart, you're done eating for the day. It's that simple.

In chapter 7 you'll see how I combine these charts with exercise goals and other tasks to help walk you through six weeks of eating and exercising to build your most beautiful body ever.

Check-Off Charts

2000 CALORIES

Wholegrain breads/starches   ❑ ❑ ❑ ❑ ❑ ❑ ❑ ❑ ❑ ❑ ❑

Vegetables   ❑ ❑ ❑ ❑   Fruits   ❑ ❑ ❑ ❑

Calcium-rich foods   ❑ ❑ ❑   Healthful fats   ❑ ❑ ❑ ❑ ❑

Protein-rich foods   ❑ ❑ ❑ ❑ ❑ ❑ ❑

1800 CALORIES

Wholegrain breads/starches   ❑ ❑ ❑ ❑ ❑ ❑ ❑ ❑ ❑ ❑

Vegetables   ❑ ❑ ❑ ❑   Fruits   ❑ ❑ ❑ ❑

Calcium-rich foods   ❑ ❑   Healthful fats   ❑ ❑ ❑ ❑

Protein-rich foods   ❑ ❑ ❑ ❑ ❑ ❑ ❑

1500 CALORIES

Wholegrain breads/starches   ❑ ❑ ❑ ❑ ❑ ❑ ❑ ❑

Vegetables   ❑ ❑ ❑   Fruits   ❑ ❑ ❑

Calcium-rich foods   ❑ ❑   Healthful fats   ❑ ❑ ❑

Protein-rich foods   ❑ ❑ ❑ ❑ ❑ ❑

1200 CALORIES

Wholegrain breads/starches   ❑ ❑ ❑ ❑ ❑ ❑

Vegetables   ❑ ❑ ❑   Fruits   ❑ ❑ ❑

Calcium-rich foods   ❑ ❑   Healthful fats   ❑ ❑ ❑

Protein-rich foods   ❑ ❑ ❑ ❑

1000 CALORIES

Wholegrain breads/starches   ❑ ❑ ❑ ❑ ❑

Vegetables   ❑ ❑ ❑   Fruits   ❑ ❑ ❑

Calcium-rich foods   ❑ ❑   Healthful fats   ❑

Protein-rich foods   ❑ ❑ ❑ ❑

2000-CALORIE SAMPLE MENU FOR ONE DAY

Breakfast

Two 3-inch whole wheat pancakes topped with 2 tablespoons light syrup and 1 cup sliced strawberries

1 cup nonfat milk

6 ounces grapefruit juice

Snack

1 apple spread with 2 tablespoons almond butter

1 cup hot herb tea with peppermint

Lunch

1 cup stir-fry tofu and snow peas over 1 cup whole wheat soba noodles

1 cup Chinese cabbage salad with 1 tablespoon nonfat vinaigrette dressing

1 fortune cookie

Snack

1.5 ounces chocolate-covered raisins

Sparkling water with lime

Dinner

4 ounces grilled sirloin steak

1 medium baked potato topped with 3/4 cup nonfat yogurt

1 cup steamed green beans

1 cup blueberries drizzled with 1 tablespoon chocolate sauce

2000 calories; 105 grams protein; 25 percent fat calories

(continues)

1800-CALORIE SAMPLE MENU FOR ONE DAY

Breakfast

1 whole egg and 2 egg whites, scrambled

1 whole grain English muffin spread with 2 teaspoons reduced-fat margarine

1 cup berries

Snack

1.5 ounces trail mix (soy nuts, dried mango, nectarines)

8 ounces lemon iced tea

Lunch

2 slices nine-grain bread spread with 3 ounces tuna mixed with chopped celery and 1 tablespoon low-fat mayo

1 cup 1-percent milk

1.5 ounces pretzels (about six pretzels)

Snack

1 orange

3 Hershey Kisses

12 ounces fitness water

Dinner

1 cup brown rice mixed with 4 ounces tofu stir-fried with 1 cup green beans and onions

2 cups romaine lettuce with 1 tomato and 2 tablespoons reduced-fat olive oil dressing

2-inch-square brownie topped with 1/2 cup vanilla nonfat yogurt

1800 calories; 93 grams protein; 22 percent fat calories

1500-CALORIE SAMPLE MENU FOR ONE DAY

Breakfast

1 cup cooked oatmeal topped with $3/4$ cup skim milk, 2 teaspoons honey, and 1 tablespoon chopped almonds

1 whole orange

Snack

3 whole-wheat crackers

Lemon-flavored hot tea

Lunch

Bean burrito (tortilla, $1/2$ cup black beans, 1 ounce reduced-fat cheese, salsa)

2 cups dark green salad with 1 whole chopped tomato and 2 tablespoons fat-free dressing

Snack

1 cup plain nonfat yogurt with 1 cup fresh blueberries swirled in

1 cup iced green tea with sweetener

Dinner

3 ounces grilled swordfish

1 cup stir-fry snow peas and cauliflower

$3/4$ cup steamed brown rice

$1/2$ sliced cucumber topped with 2 tablespoons fat-free ranch dressing

2 small chocolate candies (total of $1/2$ ounce)

1500 calories; 81 grams protein; 18 percent fat calories

(continues)

1200-CALORIE SAMPLE MENU FOR ONE DAY

Breakfast

$1/2$ whole wheat pita, toasted and spread with 1 tablespoon jam

1 cup nonfat yogurt topped with 1 medium kiwi, sliced

Snack

3 dried apricot halves

6 ounces vegetable juice

Lunch

1 cup bean soup

1 slice oat bread spread with 1 tablespoon nonfat margarine

1 cup spinach salad with 1 tablespoon nonfat dressing

Snack

$3/4$ cup nonfat milk

1 2-inch chocolate chip cookie

Dinner

$3/4$ cup whole wheat pasta topped with $1/2$ cup red sauce with 3 ounces clams

1 cup steamed summer squash sprinkled with 1 tablespoon grated Parmesan cheese

6 animal crackers dipped in 1 tablespoon hot fudge

1200 calories; 70 grams protein; 15 percent fat calories

1000-CALORIE SAMPLE MENU FOR ONE DAY

Breakfast

3/4 cup bran flakes topped with 1/2 cup blueberries and 1 cup skim milk

Snack

1 orange

12 ounces iced tea

Lunch

2 cups spinach greens tossed with 2 tablespoons fat-free Caesar dressing

3 ounces grilled chicken

1 slice toasted whole wheat sourdough bread drizzled with 1 teaspoon olive oil

1 kiwi fruit, sliced

Snack

1 cup air-popped popcorn

Dinner

1 cup vegetable soup

1/2 cup nonfat frozen yogurt topped with 2 tablespoons chocolate syrup

1000 calories; 56 grams protein; 25 percent fat calories

6

working up a sweat

Pairing your ball workout with aerobic exercise
helps you achieve faster results

Early humans worked for their food, chasing and gathering every
calorie they consumed. That simple historic fact accounts for many
of the bulging tummies and protruding rear ends in modern America.

Although our lifestyles have changed dramatically from our cave-
dwelling days, the genes that govern our metabolisms are the same.
Therefore, even though food in America is plentiful and no farther
away than the fridge or a drive-thru window, our bodies continue to
save every excess calorie and store it as though fat were still a life-sav-
ing substance. In short, the body's antique operating system hasn't
caught up with the less active way we live today.

To stay healthy, we must make the effort to incorporate more physical activity into our lives. By doing so, we can trick our bodies into
thinking that food is plentiful. All the extra movements we make will
feel like hunting and gathering.

This is why to fully make over your body—particularly if you want
to lose excess pounds—you must add cardiovascular exercise to the
formula. Your ball exercises will help tone your muscles and increase
their strength. Only cardiovascular exercise, however, will trick your
metabolism into releasing all that stored fat.

Also called aerobic exercise, cardiovascular (cardio) exercise increases your breathing and heart rate, conditioning your lungs and heart. Types of cardio exercise include power walking, jogging, tennis, cycling, and soccer, among others.

In addition to providing a number of healthful benefits, cardiovascular exercise burns off excess calories. Every mile you run or walk burns up to 100 calories, which is the equivalent of one slice of whole-grain bread with a tablespoon of jam.

In addition, your metabolism stays high for some time after you work out, boosting the number of calories you burn during later activities such as showering and eating dinner. Aerobic exercise also helps your body burn fat more easily. As you become more fit, special fat-burning enzymes increase in amount and activity and help your body mobilize fat faster. Regular doses of cardio also encourage your body to redistribute fat into your muscles for easy access during activity.

The end result: You burn a higher proportion of fat during exercise *and* during rest.

Regular cardiovascular exercise also helps regulate the appetite and is a wonderful way to prevent overeating. When you become aerobically fit, your blood sugar levels, metabolites, and numerous other factors work together to tell you when and how much to eat. The result: You get hungry when your body needs calories, and you stop eating when your calorie needs are met.

People who don't exercise aerobically don't have this appetite control mechanism. They feel hungry when they don't need calories and still feel hungry even when they should feel full. They eat more than their body needs and end up storing the excess as fat.

Finally, cardiovascular exercise not only helps you lose weight, but it also helps you keep it off. Dieters who don't do cardio exercise typically regain lost weight—and then some. When you scrimp on calories but don't do aerobic exercise, you encourage fat cells to fill up. The way your body sees it, your lack of physical activity means you're not hunting or gathering, so therefore food must be scarce and you need to fill up the fat cells for insurance.

Research on people who lose and gain weight repeatedly shows that the body increases fat storage during the regain phase, and these people often put on more weight than they lost. Some researchers theorize that this overcompensation may be why the body resists further weight-loss attempts.

People who successfully keep weight off do so by exercising daily. Cardio exercise tricks the fat cells into not filling up. Instead, fat moves to the muscles for use as fuel during workouts.

It Doesn't Have to Hurt

When many women hear the word "exercise," they cringe. The word brings back bad memories of their preteen and teen years when the boys often made fun of the girls and discriminated against them by picking them last and blaming them for team mistakes.

The thought of doing exercise also may bring back bad memories of failed fitness attempts. Perhaps you *tried* step aerobics. Or you *tried* jogging. Or you *tried* spinning. Many women have tried numerous aerobic activities—and hated them all.

If you're thinking, "That's what happened to me," there's hope for you. (Even if you're thinking, "I don't dread exercise," continue to read on. I think you'll find some invigorating ways to spice up your current routine.)

Aerobic exercise shouldn't hurt. It also shouldn't be boring or monotonous. It shouldn't make you feel self-conscious.

When women hate to exercise aerobically, it's often a result of one or more of the following.

Going Too Hard, Too Fast   Think of all the television commercials and movies that glorify jogging as the quintessential exercise for getting in shape. The videos forget to tell you that going from couch potato to all-out jogger is often not only uncomfortable but also dangerous.

Although jogging is a wonderfully efficient way to burn calories, it's not the best aerobic activity for those who are out of shape. Your

Busting a Myth

Have you heard the myth that only lower intensity exercises like walking burn fat and therefore help you lose body fat?

It's just not true. What is true is that we use up proportionately more fat than carbohydrates during low-intensity exercise. It's the greater intensity exercises like hard running that expend more overall calories per minute and more fat. Very high intensity exercises, such as sprinting, burn exclusively carbs as fuel, and in the long run you still lose body fat. This occurs after the exercise ends and the muscles start to recover, which is when fat burning revs up as glycogen stores rebuild.

But that doesn't mean you should spend all of your time exercising at a high intensity. In the final analysis, you want to exercise at an intensity that you enjoy and can maintain. So, the bottom line on losing body fat: Burn more calories than you take in. Get out there and walk!

body adjusts to exercise slowly. If you currently do no exercise, start with walking for only 10 minutes a day and then slowly increase your distance and intensity. Once you can walk for 30 minutes at an arm-swinging clip, you can consider adding bursts of jogging to the mix.

That's just one reason why my suggested cardio workouts in chapter 7 all focus on walking.

Monotony   I swim. I run. I cycle. I walk my dogs. I hike. If I only did one of these activities, I would feel bored. Our brains and bodies respond well to variety. Not only that, variety makes exercise more effective by offering new challenges to our muscles.

Rather than attending the same aerobics class three times a week, try to add one or two new activities to your repertoire. Consider an early morning walk with the dog, a tandem bike ride with your husband, a night of salsa dancing, a hike at a nearby park with your girl friends, or a game of badminton or tennis with your kids. Use your imagination. Any and all movement counts as aerobic exercise.

You can also spice up each routine with new types of workouts. You might start by adding short, faster bursts into a boring routine. Warm up for 10 minutes and then perform 1- to 2-minute bursts of faster walking, running, cycling, or swimming. Turn your daily errands into workouts by walking or riding your bike to the bank, post office, and other businesses. Enjoy nature by spotting new wildlife or wildflowers. Try fun activities from childhood such as skipping.

Thinking Negatively   Numerous studies have found that women who feel confident about their exercise abilities tend to report more joy and less discomfort during exercise than do women of equal fitness levels who go into the same session with negative thoughts. Simply put, your mind can act as a powerful motivator if you feed it the right information.

Whenever you catch yourself thinking defeatist thoughts, such as "I can't do this. I'm too weak. I don't like to sweat. I don't like to move," stop them in their tracks. You might even say, "Stop it" out loud. Then replace them with the phrase, "I can do anything I set my mind to." It sounds simple, but it works. Also, it's true. If you break any task down into baby steps, you will be taking one successful step at a time toward your goal.

It Gets Easier

As you persevere, you will find that the more you exercise aerobically, the better it feels.

Over the next six weeks, your body will make numerous adaptations that help you be less breathless and feel less fatigued as you move. This is because your muscles use the oxygen that you breathe to manufacture a substance called adenosine triphosphate (ATP). ATP gives muscles the energy they need to contract. You'll notice its effect if you exercise beyond your limit. In that case your muscles may not extract enough oxygen from your blood to keep up with demands. When ATP production falls behind, you feel the burn.

As you become more fit, however, your muscles do a better job of extracting oxygen from the blood. You'll feel a boost in your aerobic capacity that allows you to exercise at a higher intensity before your body eventually falls behind on ATP production.

During the next six weeks, the *mitochondria* in your muscle cells will multiply. Mitochondria break down fat and carbohydrates, the fuel sources that, along with oxygen, produce ATP. The more *mitochondria* in a cell, the more ATP that cell will produce, helping you feel more energized during your workouts.

Finally, regular aerobic exercise boosts the number of capillaries in your body. More blood vessels means more oxygen and nutrition can get to more areas. That improves the functioning of just about every organ in your system.

Your Cardio Goal

I strongly encourage you to try walking because it is often the easiest form of cardio to stick to. However, when it comes to exercise and fat loss, walking or any other low-key exercise will do, as long as you do it! Low-intensity exercises are a good way to start a lifetime fitness program. As you become more fit, you can do more intense exercise and burn even more calories per minute.

Here are some tips for getting the most out of your workouts.

Warm Up and Cool Down   Warming up increases the temperature of your muscles and thus reduces the risk of injury when you do your exercises. Warm-ups also allow your heart to shunt blood away from the stomach and into the muscles. At the end of your exercise period, cooling down allows the heart to redirect the blood flow back to your stomach. Warm up and cool down by starting and finishing each workout session with 5 to 10 minutes of *very* low-intensity exercise. If you go for a walk, start with slower walking and then walk faster as your muscles warm up. Then do the reverse at the end of the workout session.

Start with Walking and Then Vary It   Most women find walking to be the most accessible form of exercise. You need no equipment except for a good pair of shoes, and you can do it anywhere. That's another reason that all of the suggested cardio workouts in chapter 7 include walking. Later in this chapter I offer tips on the most effective walking techniques.

Even though walking is great cardio exercise, you should try other types of activities, too. Your fitness conditioning will be better with varied exercise, as will your motivation to stick with it.

Take a moment to think back over the various types of activities you've tried. Which ones did you most enjoy simply for the sake of moving? Also, take some time to brainstorm fun, new activities you might try, including dancing or agility training with your dog.

Build Up Your Duration   If you've never exercised before, start with just 10 minutes a day. Keep adding 5 minutes of activity a week until you hit 30 to 45 minutes. My suggested cardio workouts in chapter 7 do just that.

Do Aerobic Exercise at Least Three Days a Week   Ideally, you want to move six days a week. Your ball workout will take up three days, so aim to work out aerobically for three. That will give you one day off each week to rest.

Push Yourself   For the first two weeks of the program, work out aerobically at an easy to moderate pace. After that, start trying to speed up some of your workouts. Higher-intensity walking will help burn more calories, keep you mentally entertained, and better condition your heart and lungs.

Walk This Way

As I've mentioned, my makeover program focuses on walking, mainly because it's the most accessible form of exercise available to women. In chapter 7, you'll find three sample walking workouts for each week of the program, all designed to take you from couch potato to fitter and firmer within six weeks.

Use the following tips to get the most out of your walks.

Pay Attention to Form   You'll be able to walk faster with less discomfort if you stand tall, tighten your abs, roll from heel to toe on each foot strike, and press back through your buttocks. Bend your elbows and pump your arms for an extra calorie burn, and keep your shoulders relaxed, not hunched toward your ears.

Wear Good Shoes   Don't make the mistake of pulling those old tennis shoes from the back of your closet and wearing them during your walks. Shoes lose their ability to absorb shock over time. The upper also stretches out, providing less stability for your foot.

Considering that a complete home gym can cost thousands of dollars, a good pair of walking shoes really is a small investment. Shop at an athletic shoe store. After the sales person fits you with a shoe, walk around the store to test it. Your heel shouldn't slide and your toes shouldn't pinch. Most important, the shoe should feel comfortable.

Change It Up   As I mentioned earlier, the more variety you can add to your program, the better. Walk in different locations with different people. Try a local trail one day, the mall on a rainy day, a treadmill at the gym the next, and so on.

You should now be ready to move on to the six-week body makeover. Be sure to refer back to these earlier chapters as often as needed for tips and guidance.

7

your six-week workbook

Day-by-day tips, workouts, and eating goals
to help you stay on track

Until this point, you've been learning the nuts and bolts behind the
six-week body makeover. Because everything you'll find in your
six-week workbook builds on the material you learned in chapters 1
through 6, please make sure to read those chapters thoroughly before
starting the program.

In particular, before you begin this workbook, you must:

- Buy your fitness ball and heavy balls (see pages 3–4).

- Firmly commit yourself to completing your ball workout three
  times a week (see chapter 4).

- Pinpoint the correct weight loss pyramid for your weight and
  current eating style (see pages 119–121).

- Understand the difference between smart and troublesome
  foods (see pages 111–117).

- Choose your favorite dessert and serving size (see pages
  109–110).

- Purchase your walking shoes (see page 136).

- Choose a walking route (see page 136).

- Firmly commit yourself to build up to 30 to 45 minutes of cardiovascular exercise four times a week (see chapter 6).

Your commitment is important. Throughout the workbook, I've provided numerous tips, food checklists, suggested workouts, reflective questions, and motivational tips and techniques to help eliminate the boredom and discomfort of exercise, the psychological deprivation of healthy eating, and the motivational roadblocks to sticking with a program. These tips and techniques will bring out the natural joys of healthy eating and exercising, helping you stick with your new habits for the rest of your life.

Yet all the advice in the world won't carry you over the fitness threshold without a firm commitment from you. Take a moment right now to reflect on your commitment. Does it come from deep inside? Are you doing this for you or for someone else? List all the reasons you want to get fit and healthy. Then, with those reasons in mind, sign and date the following contract:

> *I _____ (name) pledge to make fitness and*
> *healthy eating a priority by setting aside 45 minutes every*
> *day as time just for my fitness, my thoughts, and me.*
> *I will schedule this time into my day planner.*
>
> *_____ (Signature) _____ (Date)*

How It Works

This workbook will take you from day 1—couch potato—to day 42— fit and firm. Start out by keeping track of what you eat, how you feel, and what your goals are for the day. Each journal entry includes checkboxes for you to mark off what you've eaten that day based on your food pyramid. In the blank next to the checkboxes, write the suggested number of servings listed in your food pyramid plan. Then as you eat and drink, check off the foods you've eaten. For example, if you are on the 2000-calorie food pyramid, you would write "4 servings" in the blank. Then, during the day, if you have a cup of salad for lunch and some carrots as a snack, you would check off two of the four boxes. If you eat more than the recommended amount, indicate that on the page as well to keep a record of your eating habits.

The planner also provides workout plans for each day. It uses the same ball exercises and routines outlined in chapters 1 and 2. In some cases, however, I've rearranged the order of the exercises so that each workout will feel fresh and new. For example, each Monday you'll work your body in alphabetical order from abs to triceps. Each Wednesday, you'll work backward alphabetically from triceps to abs. Each Friday, you'll work opposing muscle groups. One opposing muscle group contains the biceps along the fronts of your arms and the triceps along the backs. When one opposing muscle contracts, the other stretches. Working them one after another allows you to move through your routine faster with less rest time.

Note: This program assumes that you are sedentary and starts you out with just 10 minutes of walking during week 1. If you now exercise aerobically for more than 10 minutes, start with your current level and add 5 to 10 minutes of cardio each week until you hit a total of 35 minutes. If you'd rather do another form of cardio than walking—that's great. Just make sure to do it for at least the recommended amount of time.

Let's get started.

Week One: Day 1

Many women do too much. Let your workout serve as your *time. It's just you, the ball, and your thoughts. This is your time out from other responsibilities. This is the time you do something good for yourself.*

Check off your pyramid servings:

Wholegrain breads/starches	❏ ❏ ❏ ❏ ❏ ❏ ❏ ❏ ❏ ❏	_____	servings
Vegetables	❏ ❏ ❏ ❏	_____	servings
Fruits	❏ ❏ ❏ ❏	_____	servings
Calcium-rich foods	❏ ❏ ❏	_____	servings
Protein-rich foods	❏ ❏ ❏ ❏ ❏ ❏ ❏	_____	servings
Healthful fats	❏ ❏ ❏ ❏ ❏	_____	servings

Today I ate these smarter protein, carbohydrate, fluid, and fat choices:

_____

_____

_____

_____

_____

_____

Today I ate these troublesome protein, carbohydrate, fluid, and fat choices:

_____

_____

_____

_____

_____

Tomorrow I will try to eat smarter by:

_____

_____

_____

_____

_____

_____

Today I ate this for dessert (name and amount):

_____

_____

_____

_____

_____

Day 1 Tip: *You may feel awkward during your first ball workout. The ball may slip out from under you. You may lose your balance. That's okay. Allow yourself to laugh at your foibles. Make your workout fun. Know that in a few days you'll get the hang of it.*

Day 1 Workout:

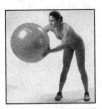

*Around the World
(page 15)*

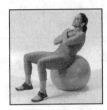

*Classic Crunches
(page 31)*

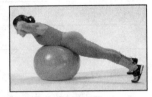

*Upper Torso Lift
(page 33)*

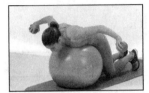

*Kneeling Back Flies
(page 35)*

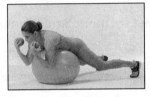

*Preacher Ball Curls
(page 36)*

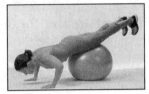

Push-Ups (page 38)

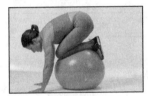

*Knee Fold-Ups
(page 40)*

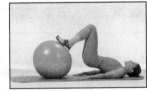

*Hamstring Curls
(page 42)*

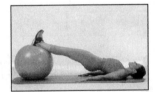

Butt Lift (page 44)

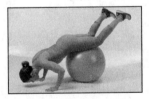

Push-Offs (page 45)

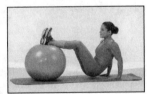

Triceps Ball Press (page 46)

Day 2

When you eat your dessert today, savor every bite. Take your dessert to a place where you have no distractions. Turn off the TV. Unplug the phone. Place a "do not disturb" sign on your office door. Smell it. Taste it. Enjoy it.

Check off your pyramid servings:

Wholegrain
  breads/starches ❑ ❑ ❑ ❑ ❑ ❑ ❑ ❑ ❑ ❑   _____ servings

Vegetables ❑ ❑ ❑ ❑   _____ servings

Fruits ❑ ❑ ❑ ❑   _____ servings

Calcium-rich foods ❑ ❑ ❑   _____ servings

Protein-rich foods ❑ ❑ ❑ ❑ ❑ ❑ ❑   _____ servings

Healthful fats ❑ ❑ ❑ ❑ ❑   _____ servings

Today I ate these smarter protein, carbohydrate, fluid, and fat choices:

_____

_____

_____

_____

_____

_____

Today I ate these troublesome protein, carbohydrate, fluid, and fat choices:

_____

_____

_____

_____

_____

_____

Tomorrow I will try to eat smarter by:

_____

_____

_____

_____

_____

Today I ate this for dessert (name and amount):

_____

_____

_____

_____

_____

Day 2 Tip: *Order yourself a new exercise outfit. The new clothes will beg you to wear them, making you look forward to your next workout.*

Day 2 Workout: *Take a 10-minute mid-morning break, remove your work shoes, and slip on your walking shoes. At a fast clip, head out of your office and down the hall. If it's a nice day, take your walk outside. Walk a few laps around the building, around the parking lot, or around the block. After 10 minutes, return to your office. In addition to conditioning your heart and burning some calories, you'll also gain more energy and focus for work!*

Day 3

You've stuck to your body makeover for three days, and I bet you're eager to see results. Try to relax. Trust the process. A caterpillar takes time to transform into a butterfly!

Check off your pyramid servings:

Wholegrain
  breads/starches ❏ ❏ ❏ ❏ ❏ ❏ ❏ ❏ ❏ ❏ _____ *servings*

Vegetables ❏ ❏ ❏ ❏   _____ *servings*

Fruits ❏ ❏ ❏ ❏   _____ *servings*

Calcium-rich foods ❏ ❏ ❏   _____ *servings*

Protein-rich foods ❏ ❏ ❏ ❏ ❏ ❏ ❏ _____ *servings*

Healthful fats ❏ ❏ ❏ ❏ ❏   _____ *servings*

Today I ate these smarter protein, carbohydrate, fluid, and fat choices:

_____

_____

_____

_____

_____

_____

Today I ate these troublesome protein, carbohydrate, fluid, and fat choices:

_____

_____

_____

_____

_____

Tomorrow I will try to eat smarter by:

_____

_____

_____

_____

_____

Today I ate this for dessert (name and amount):

_____

_____

_____

_____

_____

Day 3 Tip: *Leave your fitness ball out where you can see it. This simple visual cue can serve as a strong incentive to complete your workout.*

Day 3 Workout:

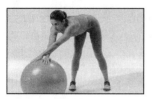

Low Body Stretch (page 16)

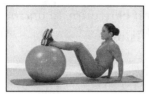

Triceps Ball Press (page 46)

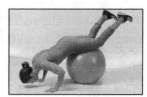

Push-Offs (page 45)

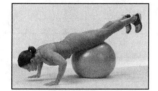

Butt Lift (page 44)

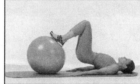

Hamstring Curls (page 42)

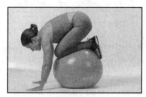

Knee Fold-Ups (page 40)

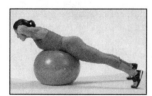

Push-Ups (page 38)

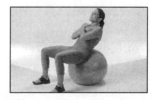

Preacher Ball Curls (page 36)

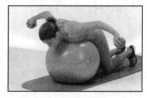

Kneeling Back Flies (page 35)

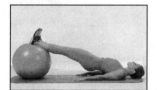

Upper Torso Lift (page 33)

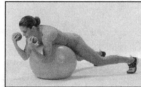

Classic Crunches (page 31)

Day 4

To overcome your fears, concentrate on the goals those fears prevent you from accomplishing.

Check off your pyramid servings:

Wholegrain
  breads/starches ❑ ❑ ❑ ❑ ❑ ❑ ❑ ❑ ❑ ❑   _____ *servings*

Vegetables ❑ ❑ ❑ ❑   _____ *servings*

Fruits ❑ ❑ ❑ ❑   _____ *servings*

Calcium-rich foods ❑ ❑ ❑   _____ *servings*

Protein-rich foods ❑ ❑ ❑ ❑ ❑ ❑ ❑   _____ *servings*

Healthful fats ❑ ❑ ❑ ❑ ❑   _____ *servings*

Today I ate these smarter protein, carbohydrate, fluid, and fat choices:

_____

_____

_____

_____

_____

_____

Today I ate these troublesome protein, carbohydrate, fluid, and fat choices:

_____

_____

_____

_____

_____

_____

Tomorrow I will try to eat smarter by:

_____

_____

_____

_____

_____

_____

Today I ate this for dessert (name and amount):

_____

_____

_____

_____

_____

Day 4 Tip: *Store your walking shoes in the car. You never know when you'll have some downtime to take a quick stroll.*

Day 4 Workout: *After work or a day watching the kids, take your partner, dog, or just yourself for a brisk 10-minute walk. Say hello to your neighbors as you stroll by. Soon you'll leave behind the tensions of the day. Your mind will be calm for a quality evening at home or with friends.*

Day 5

Your body talks to you all the time. Tune into those subtle cues, and you'll never overeat again.

Check off your pyramid servings:

*Wholegrain
 breads/starches* ❏ ❏ ❏ ❏ ❏ ❏ ❏ ❏ ❏ ❏   _____ servings

Vegetables ❏ ❏ ❏ ❏   _____ servings

Fruits ❏ ❏ ❏ ❏   _____ servings

Calcium-rich foods ❏ ❏ ❏   _____ servings

Protein-rich foods ❏ ❏ ❏ ❏ ❏ ❏ ❏   _____ servings

Healthful fats ❏ ❏ ❏ ❏ ❏   _____ servings

Today I ate these smarter protein, carbohydrate, fluid, and fat choices:

_____

_____

_____

_____

_____

_____

Today I ate these troublesome protein, carbohydrate, fluid, and fat choices:

_____

_____

_____

_____

_____

_____

Tomorrow I will try to eat smarter by:

_____

_____

_____

_____

_____

_____

Today I ate this for dessert (name and amount):

_____

_____

_____

_____

_____

Day 5 Tip: *Eat one of your meals today in total silence. Turn off the TV. Eat by yourself. Put aside any work or reading material. It's just you and your food. As the noise from the outer world subsides, the voices of your internal world will intensify. You'll hear your stomach tell you that it's full. You'll hear your taste buds tell you they've had enough. You'll hear your mind thank you for taking the time to listen.*

Day 5 Workout:

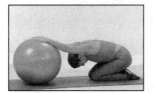

*Buddha Stretch
(page 17)*

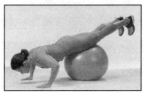

Push-Ups (page 38)

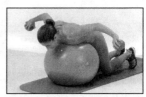

*Kneeling Back Flies
(page 35)*

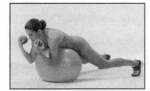

*Preacher Ball Curls
(page 36)*

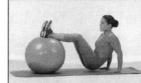

*Triceps Ball Press
(page 46)*

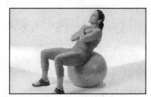

*Classic Crunches
(page 31)*

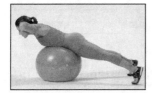

*Upper Torso Lift
(page 33)*

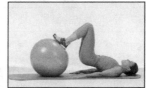

*Hamstring Curls
(page 42)*

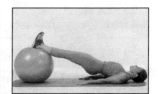

Butt Lift (page 44)

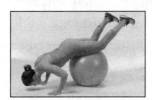

Push-Offs (page 45)

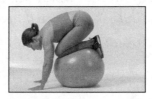

Knee Fold-Ups (page 40)

Day 6

The positive benefits of exercise far outweigh the negatives. You're burning calories. You're improving your health. You're melting away stress. You're doing something good. You're taking care of yourself.

Check off your pyramid servings:

Wholegrain breads/starches ❏ ❏ ❏ ❏ ❏ ❏ ❏ ❏ ❏ ❏	_____ servings
Vegetables ❏ ❏ ❏ ❏	_____ servings
Fruits ❏ ❏ ❏ ❏	_____ servings
Calcium-rich foods ❏ ❏ ❏	_____ servings
Protein-rich foods ❏ ❏ ❏ ❏ ❏ ❏ ❏	_____ servings
Healthful fats ❏ ❏ ❏ ❏ ❏	_____ servings

Today I ate these smarter protein, carbohydrate, fluid, and fat choices:

_____

_____

_____

_____

_____

Today I ate these troublesome protein, carbohydrate, fluid, and fat choices:

_____

_____

_____

_____

_____

Tomorrow I will try to eat smarter by:

_____

_____

_____

_____

_____

_____

Today I ate this for dessert (name and amount):

_____

_____

_____

_____

_____

_____

Day 6 Tip: *Whenever you don't feel like exercising, put on your clothes and shoes. There's something about fitness clothing that makes you want to move.*

Day 6 Workout: *Take yourself to a local park for your 10-minute walk. Explore a new place. As you walk, listen to the calls of the birds, look at the flowers and the trees, and find a world that you never before noticed.*

Day 7

Way to go! You just completed your first week. Feel good about your commitment. You've accomplished a great deal.

Check off your pyramid servings:

Wholegrain
  breads/starches ❑ ❑ ❑ ❑ ❑ ❑ ❑ ❑ ❑ ❑ _____ *servings*

Vegetables ❑ ❑ ❑ ❑ _____ *servings*

Fruits ❑ ❑ ❑ ❑ _____ *servings*

Calcium-rich foods ❑ ❑ ❑ _____ *servings*

Protein-rich foods ❑ ❑ ❑ ❑ ❑ ❑ ❑ _____ *servings*

Healthful fats ❑ ❑ ❑ ❑ ❑ _____ *servings*

Today I ate these smarter protein, carbohydrate, fluid, and fat choices:

_____

_____

_____

_____

_____

Today I ate these troublesome protein, carbohydrate, fluid, and fat choices:

_____

_____

_____

_____

_____

Tomorrow I will try to eat smarter by:

_____

_____

_____

_____

_____

_____

Today I ate this for dessert (name and amount):

_____

_____

_____

_____

_____

Day 7 Tip: *Reward yourself for a job well done. Take a warm bath. Snuggle with your dog. Find your own unique way to relax and unwind. Downtime is just as important as exercise time. During downtime your mind and body rest and rejuvenate, allowing you to face your next challenge with vigor.*

Day 7 Workout: *Today is your day off!*

Week Two: Day 8

Focus on your best intention for yourself this week. Don't aim for any more. Don't settle for any less.

Check off your pyramid servings:

Wholegrain
  breads/starches ❏ ❏ ❏ ❏ ❏ ❏ ❏ ❏ ❏ ❏   _____ servings

Vegetables ❏ ❏ ❏ ❏   _____ servings

Fruits ❏ ❏ ❏ ❏   _____ servings

Calcium-rich foods ❏ ❏ ❏   _____ servings

Protein-rich foods ❏ ❏ ❏ ❏ ❏ ❏ ❏   _____ servings

Healthful fats ❏ ❏ ❏ ❏ ❏   _____ servings

Today I ate these smarter protein, carbohydrate, fluid, and fat choices:

_____

_____

_____

_____

_____

_____

Today I ate these troublesome protein, carbohydrate, fluid, and fat choices:

_____

_____

_____

_____

_____

Tomorrow I will try to eat smarter by:

_____

_____

_____

_____

_____

Today I ate this for dessert (name and amount):

_____

_____

_____

_____

_____

Day 8 Tip: *Constantly challenge your body, and you'll constantly challenge your mind. You've done this workout before. Push yourself a little harder this week. Perhaps you can cut your rest time between sets. Or maybe you can add a few more reps.*

Day 8 Workout:

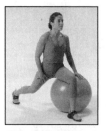
Seated Leg Stretch (page 18)

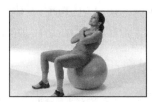
Classic Crunches (page 31)

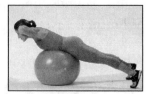
Upper Torso Lift (page 33)

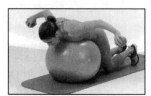
Kneeling Back Flies (page 35)

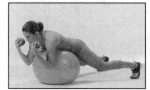
Preacher Ball Curls (page 36)

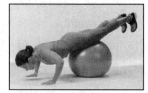
Push-Ups (page 38)

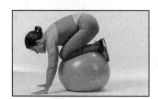
Knee Fold-Ups (page 40)

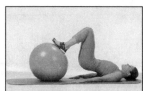
Hamstring Curls (page 42)

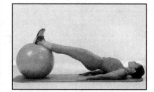
Butt Lift (page 44)

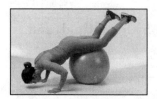
Push-Offs (page 45)

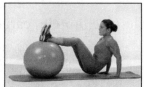
Triceps Ball Press (page 46)

Day 9

*The world presents us with endless possibilities. What new
sights, sounds, and smells do you notice during your walks?
What new tastes do you discover as you plan your meals?*

Check off your pyramid servings:

Wholegrain
 breads/starches ❑ ❑ ❑ ❑ ❑ ❑ ❑ ❑ ❑ ❑ _____ servings

Vegetables ❑ ❑ ❑ ❑ _____ servings

Fruits ❑ ❑ ❑ ❑ _____ servings

Calcium-rich foods ❑ ❑ ❑ _____ servings

Protein-rich foods ❑ ❑ ❑ ❑ ❑ ❑ ❑ _____ servings

Healthful fats ❑ ❑ ❑ ❑ ❑ _____ servings

Today I ate these smarter protein, carbohydrate, fluid, and fat
choices:

_____

_____

_____

_____

_____

_____

Today I ate these troublesome protein, carbohydrate, fluid, and
fat choices:

_____

_____

_____

_____

_____

_____

Tomorrow I will try to eat smarter by:

_____

_____

_____

_____

_____

_____

Today I ate this for dessert (name and amount):

_____

_____

_____

_____

_____

_____

Day 9 Tip: *For every negative thought that pops into your brain ("I hate exercise," "I have no willpower"), replace it with a positive one ("I can do the ball workout anywhere," "I eat well most of the time"). Positive thoughts help fuel positive actions, whereas negative thoughts derail your motivation.*

Day 9 Workout: *Walk for a total of 15 minutes today. Split up your walk by completing 5 minutes first thing in the morning, 5 more during your lunch break, and 5 in the early evening.*

Day 10

Don't feel selfish about placing your fitness needs above other responsibilities. You can't offer your best to others unless you first offer your best to yourself.

Check off your pyramid servings:

Wholegrain *breads/starches* ❑ ❑ ❑ ❑ ❑ ❑ ❑ ❑ ❑ ❑	_____	servings
Vegetables ❑ ❑ ❑ ❑	_____	servings
Fruits ❑ ❑ ❑ ❑	_____	servings
Calcium-rich foods ❑ ❑ ❑	_____	servings
Protein-rich foods ❑ ❑ ❑ ❑ ❑ ❑ ❑	_____	servings
Healthful fats ❑ ❑ ❑ ❑ ❑	_____	servings

Today I ate these smarter protein, carbohydrate, fluid, and fat choices:

_____

_____

_____

_____

_____

Today I ate these troublesome protein, carbohydrate, fluid, and fat choices:

_____

_____

_____

_____

_____

Tomorrow I will try to eat smarter by:

_____

_____

_____

_____

_____

_____

Today I ate this for dessert (name and amount):

_____

_____

_____

_____

_____

_____

Day 10 Tip: *Make exercise time a social time. Meet a girlfriend whom you rarely see for a walk at a park. Talk about anything and everything as you traverse the trails. Soon, you won't see walking as "exercise," you'll see it as social time.*

Day 10 Workout:

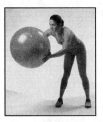

Around the World
(page 15)

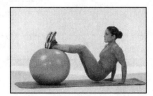

Triceps Ball Press
(page 46)

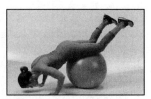

Push-Offs (page 45)

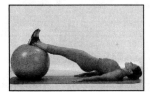

Butt Lift (page 44)

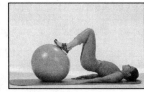

Hamstring Curls
(page 42)

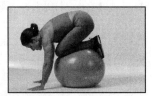

Knee Fold-Ups
(page 40)

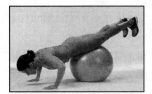

Push-Ups (page 38)

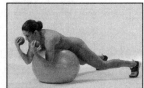

Preacher Ball Curls
(page 36)

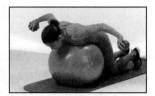

Kneeling Back Flies
(page 35)

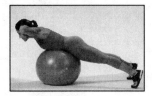

Upper Torso Lift
(page 33)

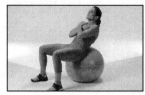

Classic Crunches (page 31)

Day 11

Your inner athlete is blooming. Talk to her. Tell her that you're sorry you kept her bottled up for so many years.

Check off your pyramid servings:

Wholegrain
  breads/starches ❏ ❏ ❏ ❏ ❏ ❏ ❏ ❏ ❏ ❏   _____ *servings*

Vegetables ❏ ❏ ❏ ❏   _____ *servings*

Fruits ❏ ❏ ❏ ❏   _____ *servings*

Calcium-rich foods ❏ ❏ ❏   _____ *servings*

Protein-rich foods ❏ ❏ ❏ ❏ ❏ ❏ ❏   _____ *servings*

Healthful fats ❏ ❏ ❏ ❏ ❏   _____ *servings*

Today I ate these smarter protein, carbohydrate, fluid, and fat choices:

_____

_____

_____

_____

_____

_____

Today I ate these troublesome protein, carbohydrate, fluid, and fat choices:

_____

_____

_____

_____

_____

Tomorrow I will try to eat smarter by:

_____

_____

_____

_____

_____

_____

Today I ate this for dessert (name and amount):

_____

_____

_____

_____

_____

Day 11 Tip: *Buy a pedometer, an inexpensive device that keeps track of how many steps you take. Sold at most sporting goods stores, these simple gadgets can encourage you to find new ways, times, and places to take your walk as you attempt to increase the number of steps over the number you did yesterday.*

Day 11 Workout: *Take yourself on a 15-minute "errand walk." Bring along a stop watch and time yourself as you walk to the post office, the bank, the hardware store, and so on. Stop the watch whenever you must stand still and start it when you begin to move again. Try to total 15 minutes of actual walking time on your errands walk.*

Day 12

Notice and celebrate every new task you complete with your stronger body, especially the tasks you once thought impossible. Strength and independence go hand in hand.

Check off your pyramid servings:

Wholegrain
  breads/starches ❑ ❑ ❑ ❑ ❑ ❑ ❑ ❑ ❑ ❑ _____ servings

Vegetables ❑ ❑ ❑ ❑ _____ servings

Fruits ❑ ❑ ❑ ❑ _____ servings

Calcium-rich foods ❑ ❑ ❑ _____ servings

Protein-rich foods ❑ ❑ ❑ ❑ ❑ ❑ ❑ _____ servings

Healthful fats ❑ ❑ ❑ ❑ ❑ _____ servings

Today I ate these smarter protein, carbohydrate, fluid, and fat choices:

_____

_____

_____

_____

_____

_____

Today I ate these troublesome protein, carbohydrate, fluid, and fat choices:

_____

_____

_____

_____

_____

_____

Tomorrow I will try to eat smarter by:

_____

_____

_____

_____

_____

Today I ate this for dessert (name and amount):

_____

_____

_____

_____

_____

Day 12 Tip: *Next time you grocery shop, buy a fruit or vegetable that you've never eaten before. If you're unsure how to prepare it, ask your grocer for suggestions. You may be surprised at how delicious many exotic foods are.*

Day 12 Workout:

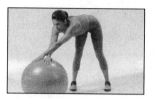
Low Body Stretch (page 16)

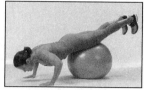
Push-Ups (page 38)

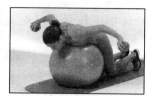
Kneeling Back Flies (page 35)

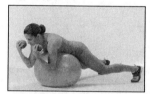
Preacher Ball Curls (page 36)

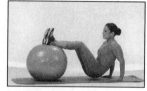
Triceps Ball Press (page 46)

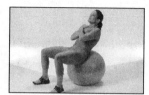
Classic Crunches (page 31)

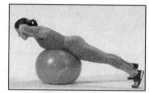
Upper Torso Lift (page 33)

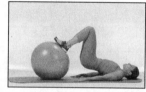
Hamstring Curls (page 42)

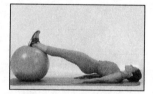
Butt Lift (page 44)

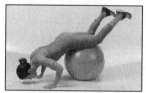
Push-Offs (page 45)

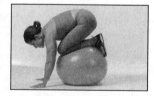
Knee Fold-Ups (page 40)

Day 13

If you believe in yourself, you can do anything.

Check off your pyramid servings:

Wholegrain
  breads/starches ❑ ❑ ❑ ❑ ❑ ❑ ❑ ❑ ❑ ❑   _____ servings

Vegetables ❑ ❑ ❑ ❑   _____ servings

Fruits ❑ ❑ ❑ ❑   _____ servings

Calcium-rich foods ❑ ❑ ❑   _____ servings

Protein-rich foods ❑ ❑ ❑ ❑ ❑ ❑ ❑   _____ servings

Healthful fats ❑ ❑ ❑ ❑ ❑   _____ servings

Today I ate these smarter protein, carbohydrate, fluid, and fat choices:

_____

_____

_____

_____

_____

Today I ate these troublesome protein, carbohydrate, fluid, and fat choices:

_____

_____

_____

_____

_____

Tomorrow I will try to eat smarter by:

_____

_____

_____

_____

_____

Today I ate this for dessert (name and amount):

_____

_____

_____

_____

_____

Day 13 Tip: *Exercise first thing in the morning. When you place fitness first on your daily "to-do" list, you're more likely to get it done. When you place it farther down the list, you run the risk of other demands taking precedence and squeezing out your fitness time.*

Day 13 Workout: *Try a 15-minute problem-solving walk. Do you have a frustrating issue at work or an ongoing battle with your teenager? Take the problem for a walk. Mull it over as you pump your arms and move your legs. By the time you return, you may have an answer.*

Day 14

Congratulations! You've successfully completed two weeks of your new fitness plan. Celebrate the new you.

Check off your pyramid servings:

Wholegrain
   breads/starches ❏ ❏ ❏ ❏ ❏ ❏ ❏ ❏ ❏ ❏ _____ *servings*

Vegetables ❏ ❏ ❏ ❏ _____ *servings*

Fruits ❏ ❏ ❏ ❏ _____ *servings*

Calcium-rich foods ❏ ❏ ❏ _____ *servings*

Protein-rich foods ❏ ❏ ❏ ❏ ❏ ❏ ❏ _____ *servings*

Healthful fats ❏ ❏ ❏ ❏ ❏ _____ *servings*

Today I ate these smarter protein, carbohydrate, fluid, and fat choices:

_____

_____

_____

_____

_____

_____

Today I ate these troublesome protein, carbohydrate, fluid, and fat choices:

_____

_____

_____

_____

_____

_____

Tomorrow I will try to eat smarter by:

_____

_____

_____

_____

_____

_____

Today I ate this for dessert (name and amount):

_____

_____

_____

_____

_____

_____

Day 14 Tip: *Most restaurant portions contain more food than we normally eat. When you eat out, ask the waiter to serve you a "half portion" of your entrée. If the restaurant doesn't offer half-portion meals, opt for two appetizers, perhaps a salad and a shrimp cocktail. Or, ask the waiter to bring a take-out container along with your order. By immediately placing half your entrée in the container, you avoid the temptation to overeat.*

Day 14 Workout: *Today is your day off. Indulge in some rest time for both your body and your mind. Relax in a hammock. Read that book you never get around to reading. Take some time just for you. You deserve it.*

Week Three: Day 15

We tend to think such horrible thoughts about the condition of our bodies, thoughts that undermine our fitness and weight-loss efforts. Yet our bodies do so much for us. Compliment your body today. Learn to appreciate it.

Check off your pyramid servings:

Wholegrain breads/starches ❏ ❏ ❏ ❏ ❏ ❏ ❏ ❏ ❏ ❏	_____ servings
Vegetables ❏ ❏ ❏ ❏	_____ servings
Fruits ❏ ❏ ❏ ❏	_____ servings
Calcium-rich foods ❏ ❏ ❏	_____ servings
Protein-rich foods ❏ ❏ ❏ ❏ ❏ ❏ ❏	_____ servings
Healthful fats ❏ ❏ ❏ ❏ ❏	_____ servings

Today I ate these smarter protein, carbohydrate, fluid, and fat choices:

_____

_____

_____

_____

_____

_____

Today I ate these troublesome protein, carbohydrate, fluid, and fat choices:

_____

_____

_____

_____

_____

_____

Tomorrow I will try to eat smarter by:

_____

_____

_____

_____

_____

_____

Today I ate this for dessert (name and amount):

_____

_____

_____

_____

_____

_____

Day 15 Tip: *Take a favorite fattening recipe and slim it down. If you like meatloaf, try adding vegetables or grains to extend the meat. Or switch to a lower fat cheese for lasagna. With a little creativity, you can enjoy all your old favorites without the excess calories—and the excess guilt.*

Day 15 Workout:

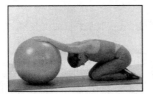

Buddha Stretch
(page 17)

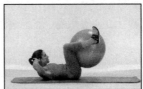

Ball Crunches
(page 47)

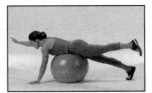

X Marks the Spot
(page 48)

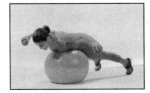

Stomach Back Flies
(page 49)

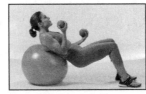

Bridge-Back Curls
(page 51)

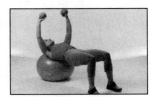

Chest Flies
(page 52)

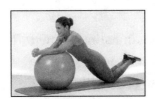

Kneeling Layouts
(page 53)

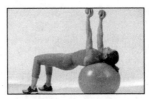

Drop Squats (page 54)

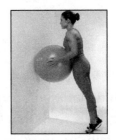

Calf Raises (page 55)

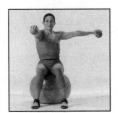

Right-Angle Lateral
Lifts (page 56)

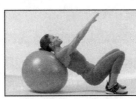

Bridge Triceps Press
(page 58)

Day 16

Celebrate every baby step on your makeover journey. You've worked hard for this.

Check off your pyramid servings:

Wholegrain
  breads/starches ❑ ❑ ❑ ❑ ❑ ❑ ❑ ❑ ❑ ❑ _____ *servings*

Vegetables ❑ ❑ ❑ ❑ _____ *servings*

Fruits ❑ ❑ ❑ ❑ _____ *servings*

Calcium-rich foods ❑ ❑ ❑ _____ *servings*

Protein-rich foods ❑ ❑ ❑ ❑ ❑ ❑ ❑ _____ *servings*

Healthful fats ❑ ❑ ❑ ❑ ❑ _____ *servings*

Today I ate these smarter protein, carbohydrate, fluid, and fat choices:

_____

_____

_____

_____

_____

_____

Today I ate these troublesome protein, carbohydrate, fluid, and fat choices:

_____

_____

_____

_____

_____

_____

Tomorrow I will try to eat smarter by:

_____

_____

_____

_____

_____

_____

Today I ate this for dessert (name and amount):

_____

_____

_____

_____

_____

_____

Day 16 Tip: *Sit on your exercise ball whenever you get the chance. Sit on it while watching TV or chatting on the phone. Periodically use it as your desk chair. Bounce on it while you watch your kids play in the yard. It's amazing how such a simple activity can effectively tone your midsection.*

Day 16 Workout: *Try to walk for 20 continuous minutes today. Go slowly for 10 minutes while your body warms up. During the middle 5 minutes of the walk, pick up your pace. Pump those arms and press through your butt as you propel yourself forward. Yes, you should feel your heart and breathing rate increase. Slow down for the last 5 minutes and allow your heart and breathing rate to return to normal.*

Day 17

Whenever you feel your motivation wane, take time out. Sit quietly and think about why you started this makeover in the first place. Are you doing it for you or to impress someone else? True motivation comes deep from within, from knowing that you're worth the struggle. Stop trying to look good for others. Start looking and feeling good for yourself.

Check off your pyramid servings:

Wholegrain breads/starches ❏ ❏ ❏ ❏ ❏ ❏ ❏ ❏ ❏ ❏ _____ servings

Vegetables ❏ ❏ ❏ ❏ _____ servings

Fruits ❏ ❏ ❏ ❏ _____ servings

Calcium-rich foods ❏ ❏ ❏ _____ servings

Protein-rich foods ❏ ❏ ❏ ❏ ❏ ❏ ❏ _____ servings

Healthful fats ❏ ❏ ❏ ❏ ❏ _____ servings

Today I ate these smarter protein, carbohydrate, fluid, and fat choices:

_____

_____

_____

_____

_____

Today I ate these troublesome protein, carbohydrate, fluid, and fat choices:

_____

_____

_____

_____

Tomorrow I will try to eat smarter by:

_____

_____

_____

_____

_____

_____

Today I ate this for dessert (name and amount):

_____

_____

_____

_____

_____

Day 17 Tip: *Have you cheated yet? Actually, that's a trick question. There's no such thing as "cheating" on this body makeover program. Whenever you find yourself cutting a walk short, putting your ball workout off until "later," or eating more dessert than you planned, don't beat yourself up. Remember: Guilt drags you down and zaps your motivation even more.*

Rather, take a look at the reasons behind your actions. Did you get enough sleep last night? Were you eating to soothe away stress? This type of self-examination will help you learn to overcome similar roadblocks in the future. You may want to jot down how you felt during these "off" times so you can avoid a relapse.

Day 17 Workout:

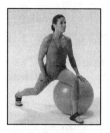

Seated Leg Stretch (page 18)

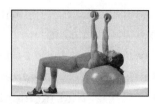

Bridge Triceps Press (page 58)

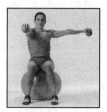

Right-Angle Lateral Lifts (page 56)

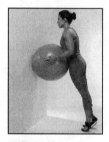

Calf Raises (page 55)

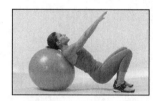

Drop Squats (page 54)

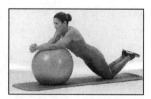

Kneeling Layouts (page 53)

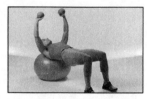

Chest Flies (page 52)

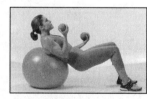

Bridge-Back Curls (page 51)

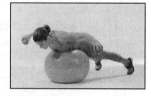

Stomach Back Flies (page 49)

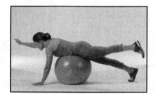

X Marks the Spot (page 48)

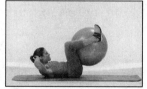

Ball Crunches (page 47)

Day 18

Sometimes you bring heavy emotional baggage with you to your workout. Your baggage may come in the form of worries ("Will I bounce a check this month?" "Why is Billy doing so poorly in school?" "How come my boyfriend hasn't called?"). Relish the moment during your workout when you drop those bags and leave them behind. Believe me, that moment always comes.

Check off your pyramid servings:

Wholegrain breads/starches ❑ ❑ ❑ ❑ ❑ ❑ ❑ ❑ ❑ ❑	_____ servings
Vegetables ❑ ❑ ❑ ❑	_____ servings
Fruits ❑ ❑ ❑ ❑	_____ servings
Calcium-rich foods ❑ ❑ ❑	_____ servings
Protein-rich foods ❑ ❑ ❑ ❑ ❑ ❑ ❑	_____ servings
Healthful fats ❑ ❑ ❑ ❑ ❑	_____ servings

Today I ate these smarter protein, carbohydrate, fluid, and fat choices:

_____.

_____

_____

_____

_____

Today I ate these troublesome protein, carbohydrate, fluid, and fat choices:

_____

_____

_____

_____

_____

Tomorrow I will try to eat smarter by:

_____

_____

_____

_____

_____

_____

Today I ate this for dessert (name and amount):

_____

_____

_____

_____

_____

_____

Day 18 Tip: *You know those jeans, the ones in the back of your closet that you won't throw out because they used to look so good on you, the ones you haven't worn in years since you gained the weight? Take them out. Place them in plain view. Every once in a while, try them on. As the weeks progress, those jeans will seem more and more roomy.*

Day 18 Workout: *Split up your walk today, doing a brisk 10 minutes in the morning and another brisk 10 just after work. Warm up for each with 2 to 3 minutes of easy strolling. Then pick up the pace for 6 minutes and cool down with a slower pace for the last few minutes.*

Day 19

Every time you exercise, you do something good for yourself. You help extend the life of your heart, lungs, bones, joints, and muscles, allowing you to be a better friend, mother, and employee in the years to come.

Check off your pyramid servings:

Wholegrain breads/starches ❑ ❑ ❑ ❑ ❑ ❑ ❑ ❑ ❑ ❑	_____	*servings*
Vegetables ❑ ❑ ❑ ❑	_____	*servings*
Fruits ❑ ❑ ❑ ❑	_____	*servings*
Calcium-rich foods ❑ ❑ ❑	_____	*servings*
Protein-rich foods ❑ ❑ ❑ ❑ ❑ ❑ ❑	_____	*servings*
Healthful fats ❑ ❑ ❑ ❑ ❑	_____	*servings*

Today I ate these smarter protein, carbohydrate, fluid, and fat choices:

_____

_____

_____

_____

_____

Today I ate these troublesome protein, carbohydrate, fluid, and fat choices:

_____

_____

_____

_____

_____

Tomorrow I will try to eat smarter by:

_____

_____

_____

_____

_____

_____

Today I ate this for dessert (name and amount):

_____

_____

_____

_____

_____

_____

Day 19 Tip: *Do a taste test today. Pick a healthful product that you've been scared to try—maybe soy cheese or veggie sausage. Buy a few brands and invite friends over for a taste test. You'll find that individual brands may taste dramatically different. Often times, choosing and continuing to eat a more healthful food is merely a matter of finding the brand you like.*

Day 19 Workout:

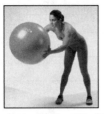

*Around the World
(page 15)*

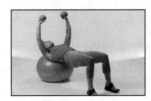

Chest Flies (page 52)

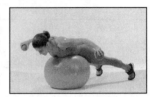

*Stomach Back Flies
(page 49)*

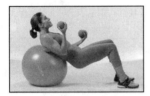

*Bridge-Back Curls
(page 51)*

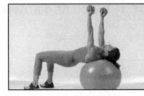

*Bridge Triceps Press
(page 58)*

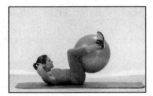

*Ball Crunches
(page 47)*

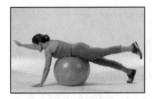

*X Marks the Spot
(page 48)*

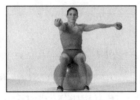

*Right-Angle Lateral
Lifts (page 56)*

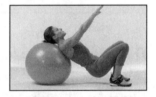

Drop Squats (page 54)

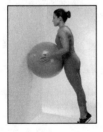

Calf Raises (page 55)

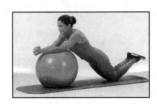

Kneeling Layouts (page 53)

Day 20

Make a game out of restaurant eating. Allow yourself naughty foods like tortilla chips, crunchy Chinese noodles, and French fries. But don't eat all of them. Set a limit before your first bite and stick to it. Enjoy your favorite foods and bolster your willpower in the process!

Check off your pyramid servings:

Wholegrain
  breads/starches ❏ ❏ ❏ ❏ ❏ ❏ ❏ ❏ ❏ ❏   _____ *servings*

Vegetables ❏ ❏ ❏ ❏   _____ *servings*

Fruits ❏ ❏ ❏ ❏   _____ *servings*

Calcium-rich foods ❏ ❏ ❏   _____ *servings*

Protein-rich foods ❏ ❏ ❏ ❏ ❏ ❏ ❏   _____ *servings*

Healthful fats ❏ ❏ ❏ ❏ ❏   _____ *servings*

Today I ate these smarter protein, carbohydrate, fluid, and fat choices:

_____

_____

_____

_____

_____

Today I ate these troublesome protein, carbohydrate, fluid, and fat choices:

_____

_____

_____

_____

_____

Tomorrow I will try to eat smarter by:

_____

_____

_____

_____

_____

_____

Today I ate this for dessert (name and amount):

_____

_____

_____

_____

_____

_____

Day 20 Tip: *Try to burn extra calories during everyday tasks. Instead of piling items at the bottom of the steps to carry up in one load, carry them one at a time. Power walk through the house as you straighten it. Walk to a co-worker's officer rather than sending e-mail. All these small tasks can add up to many extra burned calories by day's end.*

Day 20 Workout: *Wear a stopwatch today. During every snippet of free time, take a short walk. Start your watch at the beginning of your walk and stop it at the end. You might walk for 3 minutes around the parking lot as you wait for your hairdresser to show up. Or you might power walk from one department store to another while shopping at the mall. Keep a tally of the total minutes you walk. Try to get them to add up to 20 or more for the day.*

Day 21

Congratulations! You just completed three weeks of the program. Way to go!

Check off your pyramid servings:

Wholegrain
  breads/starches ❑ ❑ ❑ ❑ ❑ ❑ ❑ ❑ ❑ ❑ _____ *servings*

Vegetables ❑ ❑ ❑ ❑ _____ *servings*

Fruits ❑ ❑ ❑ ❑ _____ *servings*

Calcium-rich foods ❑ ❑ ❑ _____ *servings*

Protein-rich foods ❑ ❑ ❑ ❑ ❑ ❑ ❑ _____ *servings*

Healthful fats ❑ ❑ ❑ ❑ ❑ _____ *servings*

Today I ate these smarter protein, carbohydrate, fluid, and fat choices:

_____

_____

_____

_____

_____

_____

Today I ate these troublesome protein, carbohydrate, fluid, and fat choices:

_____

_____

_____

_____

_____

_____

Tomorrow I will try to eat smarter by:

_____

_____

_____

_____

_____

_____

Today I ate this for dessert (name and amount):

_____

_____

_____

_____

_____

_____

Day 21 Tip: *Plan your meals for the week. You might try one new recipe along with some quick-and-easy favorites like BBQ chicken or grilled fish. Make a list, check your recipes, and then head to the grocery store for the ingredients. This kind of planning will help you avoid a food emergency.*

Day 21 Workout: *Today is your day off. Take the time you would have exercised and spend it relaxing.*

Week Four: Day 22

Some say that beauty is only skin deep. I think it goes deeper, much deeper, to your very core, where your inner confidence radiates outward.

Check off your pyramid servings:

Wholegrain
  breads/starches ❏ ❏ ❏ ❏ ❏ ❏ ❏ ❏ ❏ ❏   _____ *servings*

Vegetables ❏ ❏ ❏ ❏   _____ *servings*

Fruits ❏ ❏ ❏ ❏   _____ *servings*

Calcium-rich foods ❏ ❏ ❏   _____ *servings*

Protein-rich foods ❏ ❏ ❏ ❏ ❏ ❏ ❏   _____ *servings*

Healthful fats ❏ ❏ ❏ ❏ ❏   _____ *servings*

Today I ate these smarter protein, carbohydrate, fluid, and fat choices:

_____

_____

_____

_____

_____

_____

Today I ate these troublesome protein, carbohydrate, fluid, and fat choices:

_____

_____

_____

_____

_____

_____

Tomorrow I will try to eat smarter by:

_____
_____
_____
_____
_____
_____

Today I ate this for dessert (name and amount):

_____
_____
_____
_____
_____
_____

Day 22 Tip: *Continually challenge yourself during your workouts. Meeting challenges will boost your motivation as well as your success. Start today by cutting back on the time you rest between exercises and doing more reps of each exercise than you did last week.*

Day 22 Workout:

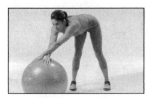

*Low Body Stretch
(page 16)*

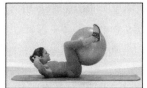

*Ball Crunches
(page 47)*

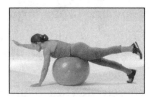

*X Marks the Spot
(page 48)*

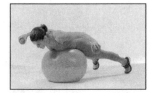

*Stomach Back Flies
(page 49)*

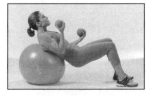

*Bridge-Back Curls
(page 51)*

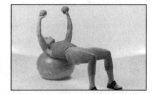

Chest Flies (page 52)

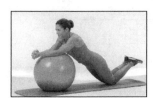

*Kneeling Layouts
(page 53)*

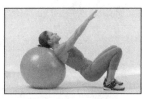

*Drop Squats
(page 54)*

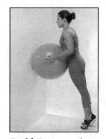

Calf Raises (page 55)

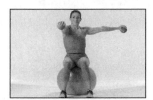

*Right-Angle Lateral
Lifts (page 56)*

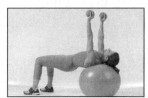

*Bridge Triceps Press
(page 58)*

Day 23

Everyone drags through a workout at one time or another. On those days when every movement feels as if you're plowing through molasses, slow down and listen.

Check off your pyramid servings:

Wholegrain
  breads/starches ❏ ❏ ❏ ❏ ❏ ❏ ❏ ❏ ❏ ❏   _____ servings

Vegetables ❏ ❏ ❏ ❏   _____ servings

Fruits ❏ ❏ ❏ ❏   _____ servings

Calcium-rich foods ❏ ❏ ❏   _____ servings

Protein-rich foods ❏ ❏ ❏ ❏ ❏ ❏ ❏   _____ servings

Healthful fats ❏ ❏ ❏ ❏ ❏   _____ servings

Today I ate these smarter protein, carbohydrate, fluid, and fat choices:

_____

_____

_____

_____

_____

Today I ate these troublesome protein, carbohydrate, fluid, and fat choices:

_____

_____

_____

_____

_____

_____

Tomorrow I will try to eat smarter by:

_____

_____

_____

_____

_____

_____

Today I ate this for dessert (name and amount):

_____

_____

_____

_____

_____

_____

Day 23 Tip: *Everyday life presents us with so many opportunities to burn extra calories. Walk every chance you get by parking at the far end of every parking lot. Also, play actively with your kids. Instead of watching them play hopscotch or tag, join them!*

Day 23 Workout: *Walk for 25 minutes today. Warm up for 5 minutes with slower walking and then pump your arms as you pick up the pace. Walk at a fast clip for 1 minute and then slow down to your normal pace for 2 minutes. Continue alternating between 1 minute of faster walking and 2 minutes of slower walking for the next 15 minutes. Cool down with 5 minutes at an easy pace.*

Day 24

See every obstacle as a challenge. Rather than allow obstacles to defeat you, rise above them by brainstorming ways you can avoid the same pitfall in the future.

Check off your pyramid servings:

Wholegrain
  breads/starches ❏ ❏ ❏ ❏ ❏ ❏ ❏ ❏ ❏ ❏   _____ servings

Vegetables ❏ ❏ ❏ ❏   _____ servings

Fruits ❏ ❏ ❏ ❏   _____ servings

Calcium-rich foods ❏ ❏ ❏   _____ servings

Protein-rich foods ❏ ❏ ❏ ❏ ❏ ❏ ❏   _____ servings

Healthful fats ❏ ❏ ❏ ❏ ❏   _____ servings

Today I ate these smarter protein, carbohydrate, fluid, and fat choices:

_____

_____

_____

_____

_____

Today I ate these troublesome protein, carbohydrate, fluid, and fat choices:

_____

_____

_____

_____

_____

Tomorrow I will try to eat smarter by:

_____

_____

_____

_____

_____

_____

Today I ate this for dessert (name and amount):

_____

_____

_____

_____

_____

_____

Day 24 Tip: *Increase your calorie burn during your ball work-out by adding short snippets of aerobic activity during your "rest" breaks. For example, try marching in place, skipping rope, or walking around the backyard between ball exercises.*

Day 24 Workout:

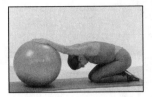

Buddha Stretch
(page 17)

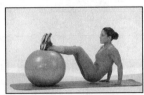

Triceps Ball Press
(page 46)

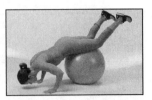

Push-Offs (page 45)

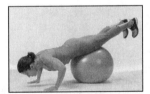

Butt Lift (page 44)

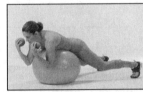

Hamstring Curls
(page 42)

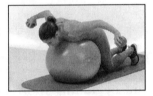

Knee Fold-Ups
(page 40)

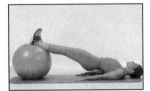

Push-Ups (page 38)

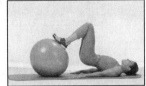

Preacher Ball Curls
(page 36)

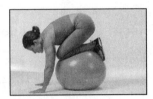

Kneeling Back Flies
(page 35)

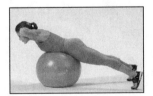

Upper Torso Lift
(page 33)

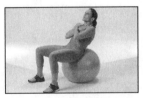

Classic Crunches (page 31)

Day 25

Have you thought about quitting? Whenever such thoughts come to mind, remind yourself that you're not a quitter. You're the type of woman who finishes what she starts.

Check off your pyramid servings:

Wholegrain
  breads/starches ❑ ❑ ❑ ❑ ❑ ❑ ❑ ❑ ❑ ❑ _____ *servings*

Vegetables ❑ ❑ ❑ ❑ _____ *servings*

Fruits ❑ ❑ ❑ ❑ _____ *servings*

Calcium-rich foods ❑ ❑ ❑ _____ *servings*

Protein-rich foods ❑ ❑ ❑ ❑ ❑ ❑ ❑ _____ *servings*

Healthful fats ❑ ❑ ❑ ❑ ❑ _____ *servings*

Today I ate these smarter protein, carbohydrate, fluid, and fat choices:

_____

_____

_____

_____

Today I ate these troublesome protein, carbohydrate, fluid, and fat choices:

_____

_____

_____

_____

Tomorrow I will try to eat smarter by:

_____

_____

_____

_____

_____

_____

Today I ate this for dessert (name and amount):

_____

_____

_____

_____

_____

_____

Day 25 Tip: *To lower the number of calories in an omelet without missing out on the rich taste, mix one real egg with two egg whites. Egg whites contain fewer calories than whole eggs, and the one yolk will add taste, vital nutrients, texture, and color to your omelet.*

Day 25 Workout: *Walk for 25 minutes today. Warm up for 5 minutes with slower walking and then pump your arms as you pick up the pace. Walk at a fast clip for 2 minutes and then resume your normal pace for 2 minutes. Continue alternating between 2 minutes of faster walking and 2 minutes of slower walking for the next 15 minutes. Cool down with 5 minutes at an easy pace.*

Day 26

Focus on the journey rather than the destination. Maintaining health, fitness, and weight is a lifelong journey, one that never ends.

Check off your pyramid servings:

Wholegrain
  breads/starches ❑ ❑ ❑ ❑ ❑ ❑ ❑ ❑ ❑ ❑ _____ *servings*

Vegetables ❑ ❑ ❑ ❑ _____ *servings*

Fruits ❑ ❑ ❑ ❑ _____ *servings*

Calcium-rich foods ❑ ❑ ❑ _____ *servings*

Protein-rich foods ❑ ❑ ❑ ❑ ❑ ❑ ❑ _____ *servings*

Healthful fats ❑ ❑ ❑ ❑ ❑ _____ *servings*

Today I ate these smarter protein, carbohydrate, fluid, and fat choices:

_____

_____

_____

_____

_____

Today I ate these troublesome protein, carbohydrate, fluid, and fat choices:

_____

_____

_____

_____

_____

Tomorrow I will try to eat smarter by:

_____

_____

_____

_____

_____

_____

Today I ate this for dessert (name and amount):

_____

_____

_____

_____

_____

_____

Day 26 Tip: *Never go to the grocery store hungry. When you do, all the foods that you normally wouldn't put in your cart just seem to jump off the shelves.*

Day 26 Workout:

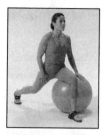

Seated Leg Stretch (page 18)

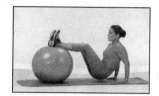

Triceps Ball Press (page 46)

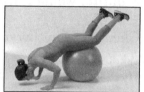

Push-Offs (page 45)

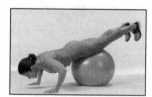

Butt Lift (page 44)

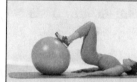

Hamstring Curls (page 42)

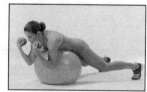

Knee Fold-Ups (page 40)

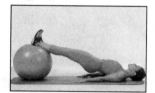

Push-Ups (page 38)

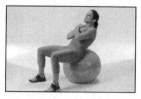

Preacher Ball Curls (page 36)

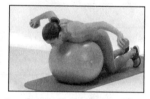

Kneeling Back Flies (page 35)

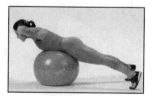

Upper Torso Lift (page 33)

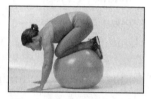

Classic Crunches (page 31)

Day 27

There's no such thing as a perfect body. Even the thinnest, most beautiful women struggle with their body image.

Check off your pyramid servings:

Wholegrain
  breads/starches ❑ ❑ ❑ ❑ ❑ ❑ ❑ ❑ ❑ ❑ _____ servings

Vegetables ❑ ❑ ❑ ❑   _____ servings

Fruits ❑ ❑ ❑ ❑   _____ servings

Calcium-rich foods ❑ ❑ ❑   _____ servings

Protein-rich foods ❑ ❑ ❑ ❑ ❑ ❑ ❑   _____ servings

Healthful fats ❑ ❑ ❑ ❑ ❑   _____ servings

Today I ate these smarter protein, carbohydrate, fluid, and fat choices:

_____

_____

_____

_____

_____

_____

Today I ate these troublesome protein, carbohydrate, fluid, and fat choices:

_____

_____

_____

_____

_____

_____

Tomorrow I will try to eat smarter by:

_____

_____

_____

_____

_____

Today I ate this for dessert (name and amount):

_____

_____

_____

_____

_____

Day 27 Tip: *Magazines taint our image of the ideal woman's body. They take a picture of an already slender supermodel and airbrush off the cellulite, smooth out the wrinkles, and sometimes use a computer to elongate the torso. The result is a photo that even the supermodel could never look like. Whenever you feel that your body doesn't quite measure up to the perfect women you see in the media, examine your measuring stick. You may be comparing yourself to a body that doesn't exist.*

Day 27 Workout: *Walk for 25 minutes today. Warm up for 5 minutes with slower walking and then pump your arms as you pick up the pace. Walk at a fast clip for 3 minutes and then resume your normal pace for 2 minutes. Continue alternating between 3 minutes of faster walking and 2 minutes of slower walking for the next 15 minutes. Cool down with 5 minutes at an easy pace.*

Day 28

*Congratulations! You just completed four weeks of the program.
Way to go!*

Check off your pyramid servings:

Wholegrain
  breads/starches ❏ ❏ ❏ ❏ ❏ ❏ ❏ ❏ ❏ ❏   _____ servings

Vegetables ❏ ❏ ❏ ❏   _____ servings

Fruits ❏ ❏ ❏ ❏   _____ servings

Calcium-rich foods ❏ ❏ ❏   _____ servings

Protein-rich foods ❏ ❏ ❏ ❏ ❏ ❏ ❏   _____ servings

Healthful fats ❏ ❏ ❏ ❏ ❏   _____ servings

Today I ate these smarter protein, carbohydrate, fluid, and fat
choices:

_____

_____

_____

_____

_____

_____

Today I ate these troublesome protein, carbohydrate, fluid, and
fat choices:

_____

_____

_____

_____

_____

Tomorrow I will try to eat smarter by:

_____

_____

_____

_____

_____

_____

Today I ate this for dessert (name and amount):

_____

_____

_____

_____

_____

Day 28 Tip: *Your rest time is just as important as your exercise time. Your muscles grow and repair themselves when you rest them between sessions. Never try to rush weight loss by strength training every day. You'll eventually experience diminishing returns.*

Day 28 Workout: *Today is your day off. Instead of exercising, treat yourself. Sign up for a massage. Relax in a hot tub. Take a nap in a hammock.*

Week Five: Day 29

Your new fit lifestyle should now be part of you. Congratulate yourself for forming new healthy habits.

Check off your pyramid servings:

Wholegrain
  breads/starches ❏ ❏ ❏ ❏ ❏ ❏ ❏ ❏ ❏ ❏ _____ *servings*

Vegetables ❏ ❏ ❏ ❏ _____ *servings*

Fruits ❏ ❏ ❏ ❏ _____ *servings*

Calcium-rich foods ❏ ❏ ❏ _____ *servings*

Protein-rich foods ❏ ❏ ❏ ❏ ❏ ❏ ❏ _____ *servings*

Healthful fats ❏ ❏ ❏ ❏ ❏ _____ *servings*

Today I ate these smarter protein, carbohydrate, fluid, and fat choices:

_____

_____

_____

_____

_____

_____

Today I ate these troublesome protein, carbohydrate, fluid, and fat choices:

_____

_____

_____

_____

_____

Tomorrow I will try to eat smarter by:

_____

_____

_____

_____

_____

Today I ate this for dessert (name and amount):

_____

_____

_____

_____

_____

Day 29 Tip: *Fish is one of the best low-calorie sources of quality protein you can eat. Especially if you eat fatty, cold water fish like salmon, you'll ingest the important omega-3 fatty acids, known to ease joint pain, give your skin a radiant glow, possibly prevent wrinkles, and generally bolster your overall health. Try to eat fish at least twice a week.*

Day 29 Workout:

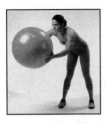

*Around the World
(page 15)*

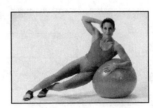

Side-Ups (page 59)

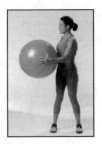

*Standing Torso Twist
(page 60)*

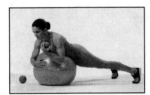

*Off-the-Ball Curls
(page 63)*

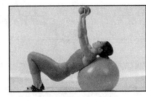

*Chest-Press Incline
(page 64)*

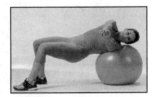

*Arm-Swing Rolls
(page 65)*

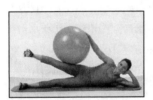

Thigh Buster (page 66)

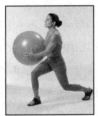

Atlas Lunge (page 68)

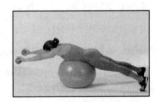

Flying Carpet (page 69)

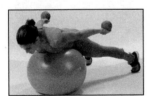

Triceps Extension (page 70)

Day 30

Core strength helps you navigate life with less effort. When your workouts feel too hard, remember that they make the rest of your life so much easier.

Check off your pyramid servings:

Wholegrain
  breads/starches ❏ ❏ ❏ ❏ ❏ ❏ ❏ ❏ ❏ ❏   _____ servings

Vegetables ❏ ❏ ❏ ❏   _____ servings

Fruits ❏ ❏ ❏ ❏   _____ servings

Calcium-rich foods ❏ ❏ ❏   _____ servings

Protein-rich foods ❏ ❏ ❏ ❏ ❏ ❏ ❏   _____ servings

Healthful fats ❏ ❏ ❏ ❏ ❏   _____ servings

Today I ate these smarter protein, carbohydrate, fluid, and fat choices:

_____

_____

_____

_____

_____

_____

Today I ate these troublesome protein, carbohydrate, fluid, and fat choices:

_____

_____

_____

_____

_____

_____

Tomorrow I will try to eat smarter by:

_____

_____

_____

_____

_____

Today I ate this for dessert (name and amount):

_____

_____

_____

_____

_____

Day 30 Tip: *Buy a cordless phone. That way you can power walk through your house as you talk to your friends.*

Day 30 Workout: *Walk for 30 minutes today. Warm up for 5 minutes with slower walking and then pump your arms as you pick up the pace. Walk at a fast clip for 4 minutes and then slow down to your normal pace for 2 minutes. Continue alternating between 4 minutes of faster walking and 2 minutes of slower walking for the next 20 minutes. Cool down with 5 minutes at an easy pace.*

Day 31

You're well on your way to meeting your goal. Your options are endless. What new goal will you set for yourself after week 6?

Check off your pyramid servings:

Wholegrain
  breads/starches ❑ ❑ ❑ ❑ ❑ ❑ ❑ ❑ ❑ ❑   _____ *servings*

Vegetables ❑ ❑ ❑ ❑   _____ *servings*

Fruits ❑ ❑ ❑ ❑   _____ *servings*

Calcium-rich foods ❑ ❑ ❑   _____ *servings*

Protein-rich foods ❑ ❑ ❑ ❑ ❑ ❑ ❑   _____ *servings*

Healthful fats ❑ ❑ ❑ ❑ ❑   _____ *servings*

Today I ate these smarter protein, carbohydrate, fluid, and fat choices:

_____

_____

_____

_____

_____

Today I ate these troublesome protein, carbohydrate, fluid, and fat choices:

_____

_____

_____

_____

_____

Tomorrow I will try to eat smarter by:

_____
_____
_____
_____
_____
_____

Today I ate this for dessert (name and amount):

_____
_____
_____
_____
_____
_____

Day 31 Tip: *Research shows that you can make an exercise more effective simply by lifting a weight more slowly. The "super slow" method works because it recruits more muscle fibers as you lift the weight without the benefit of momentum. Slow down your workout today, lifting your heavy balls slowly. You won't be able to complete as many repetitions, but you'll accomplish more.*

Day 31 Workout:

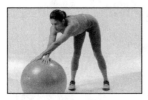

Low Body Stretch (page 16)

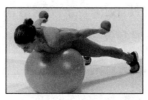

Triceps Extension (page 70)

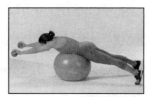

Flying Carpet (page 69)

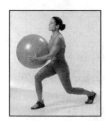

Atlas Lunge (page 68)

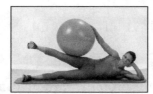

Thigh Buster (page 66)

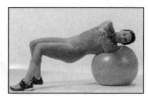

Arm-Swing Rolls (page 65)

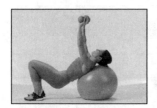

Chest-Press Incline (page 64

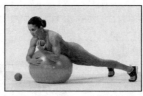

Off-the-Ball Curls (page 63)

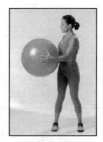

Standing Torso Twist (page 60)

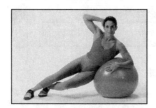

Side-Ups (page 59)

Day 32

Remember that little girl so long ago who once hated gym class? If only she could see you today!

Check off your pyramid servings:

Wholegrain
  breads/starches ❑ ❑ ❑ ❑ ❑ ❑ ❑ ❑ ❑ ❑ _____ servings

Vegetables ❑ ❑ ❑ ❑   _____ servings

Fruits ❑ ❑ ❑ ❑   _____ servings

Calcium-rich foods ❑ ❑ ❑   _____ servings

Protein-rich foods ❑ ❑ ❑ ❑ ❑ ❑ ❑   _____ servings

Healthful fats ❑ ❑ ❑ ❑ ❑   _____ servings

Today I ate these smarter protein, carbohydrate, fluid, and fat choices:

_____

_____

_____

_____

_____

_____

Today I ate these troublesome protein, carbohydrate, fluid, and fat choices:

_____

_____

_____

_____

_____

Tomorrow I will try to eat smarter by:

_____

_____

_____

_____

_____

_____

Today I ate this for dessert (name and amount):

_____

_____

_____

_____

_____

_____

Day 32 Tip: *Pay attention to all the wonderful side benefits of fitness. Sure, your program helps you look and feel great. Has it also opened up your social connections? I bet you now know most of your neighbors from power walking by their houses every other day. Fitness will open your life to an entirely new community of friends.*

Day 32 Workout: *Walk for 30 minutes today. Warm up for 5 minutes with slower walking and then pump your arms as you pick up the pace. Walk at a fast clip for 4 minutes and then slow down to your normal pace for 2 minutes. Continue alternating between 4 minutes of faster walking and 2 minutes of slower walking for the next 20 minutes. Cool down with 5 minutes at an easy pace.*

Day 33

Achieving a fit body isn't a matter of genetics. It's a matter of priorities.

Check off your pyramid servings:

Wholegrain
  breads/starches ❑ ❑ ❑ ❑ ❑ ❑ ❑ ❑ ❑ ❑   _____ *servings*

Vegetables ❑ ❑ ❑ ❑   _____ *servings*

Fruits ❑ ❑ ❑ ❑   _____ *servings*

Calcium-rich foods ❑ ❑ ❑   _____ *servings*

Protein-rich foods ❑ ❑ ❑ ❑ ❑ ❑ ❑   _____ *servings*

Healthful fats ❑ ❑ ❑ ❑ ❑   _____ *servings*

Today I ate these smarter protein, carbohydrate, fluid, and fat choices:

_____

_____

_____

_____

_____

_____

Today I ate these troublesome protein, carbohydrate, fluid, and fat choices:

_____

_____

_____

_____

_____

Tomorrow I will try to eat smarter by:

_____

_____

_____

_____

_____

Today I ate this for dessert (name and amount):

_____

_____

_____

_____

_____

Day 33 Tip: *Many women eat more than 3 to 4 ounces of red meat in one sitting. Part of the problem is that a typical steak weighs 6 to 8 ounces. To cut back on extra fat and calories from red meat, slice it up and use it as one ingredient rather than the entire main course. Try a red meat stir-fry or a beef and bean burrito, for example.*

Day 33 Workout:

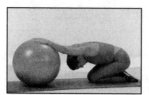

Buddha Stretch
(page 17)

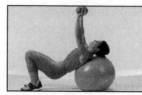

Chest-Press Incline
(page 64)

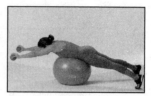

Flying Carpet
(page 69)

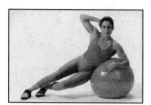

Side-Ups (page 59)

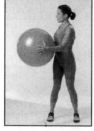

Standing Torso Twist
(page 60)

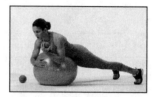

Off-the-Ball Curls
(page 63)

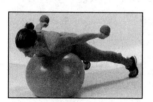

Triceps Extension
(page 70)

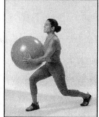

Atlas Lunge (page 68)

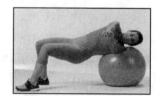

Arm-Swing Rolls
(page 65)

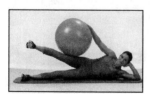

Thigh Buster (page 66)

Day 34

Sometimes you may not feel like walking during the first 10 minutes. After 10 minutes, you may not want to stop.

Check off your pyramid servings:

Wholegrain
  breads/starches ❏ ❏ ❏ ❏ ❏ ❏ ❏ ❏ ❏ ❏ _____ *servings*

Vegetables ❏ ❏ ❏ ❏ _____ *servings*

Fruits ❏ ❏ ❏ ❏ _____ *servings*

Calcium-rich foods ❏ ❏ ❏ _____ *servings*

Protein-rich foods ❏ ❏ ❏ ❏ ❏ ❏ ❏ _____ *servings*

Healthful fats ❏ ❏ ❏ ❏ ❏ _____ *servings*

Today I ate these smarter protein, carbohydrate, fluid, and fat choices:

_____

_____

_____

_____

_____

_____

Today I ate these troublesome protein, carbohydrate, fluid, and fat choices:

_____

_____

_____

_____

_____

_____

Tomorrow I will try to eat smarter by:

_____

_____

_____

_____

_____

Today I ate this for dessert (name and amount):

_____

_____

_____

_____

_____

_____

_____

Day 34 Tip: *Schedule your fitness time in your day planner along with all your other meetings and daily tasks. Even pencil it in several days in advance.*

Day 34 Workout: *Walk for 30 minutes today. Warm up for 5 minutes with slower walking and then pump your arms as you pick up the pace. Walk at a fast clip for 4 minutes and then slow down to your normal pace for 2 minutes. Continue alternating between 4 minutes of faster walking and 2 minutes of slower walking for the next 20 minutes. Cool down with 5 minutes at an easy pace.*

Day 35

*Congratulations! You just completed five weeks of the program.
Way to go!*

Check off your pyramid servings:

*Wholegrain
  breads/starches* ❑ ❑ ❑ ❑ ❑ ❑ ❑ ❑ ❑ ❑ _____ *servings*

Vegetables ❑ ❑ ❑ ❑ _____ *servings*

Fruits ❑ ❑ ❑ ❑ _____ *servings*

Calcium-rich foods ❑ ❑ ❑ _____ *servings*

Protein-rich foods ❑ ❑ ❑ ❑ ❑ ❑ ❑ _____ *servings*

Healthful fats ❑ ❑ ❑ ❑ ❑ _____ *servings*

Today I ate these smarter protein, carbohydrate, fluid, and fat choices:

_____

_____

_____

_____

_____

_____

Today I ate these troublesome protein, carbohydrate, fluid, and fat choices:

_____

_____

_____

_____

_____

_____

Tomorrow I will try to eat smarter by:

_____

_____

_____

_____

_____

_____

Today I ate this for dessert (name and amount):

_____

_____

_____

_____

_____

_____

Day 35 Tip: *Reward yourself for all your hard work by signing up for a massage. In addition to making you feel wonderful and helping you relax, a massage will help break up knots or tight spots in your muscles, helping you exercise with more ease.*

Day 35 Workout: *Today is your day off. Take the time you would normally have spent exercising and use it as time to relax.*

Week Six: Day 36

Many people remain unfit because they are scared of change.
Think of how many changes you've made during the past month.
With so much change under your belt, what else will you decide
to accomplish?

Check off your pyramid servings:

Wholegrain
  breads/starches ❏ ❏ ❏ ❏ ❏ ❏ ❏ ❏ ❏ ❏   _____ servings

Vegetables ❏ ❏ ❏ ❏   _____ servings

Fruits ❏ ❏ ❏ ❏   _____ servings

Calcium-rich foods ❏ ❏ ❏   _____ servings

Protein-rich foods ❏ ❏ ❏ ❏ ❏ ❏ ❏   _____ servings

Healthful fats ❏ ❏ ❏ ❏ ❏   _____ servings

Today I ate these smarter protein, carbohydrate, fluid, and fat
choices:

_____

_____

_____

_____

_____

Today I ate these troublesome protein, carbohydrate, fluid, and
fat choices:

_____

_____

_____

_____

_____

Tomorrow I will try to eat smarter by:

_____

_____

_____

_____

_____

_____

Today I ate this for dessert (name and amount):

_____

_____

_____

_____

_____

Day 36 Tip: *If you tend to overeat when you snack, opt for snacks that come in individual servings. Try a small carton of yogurt or cottage cheese or even a small package of peanut butter crackers.*

Day 36 Workout:

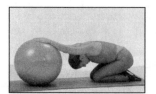

Buddha Stretch (page 17)

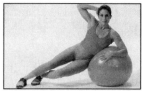

Side-Ups (page 59)

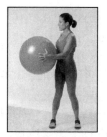

Standing Torso Twist (page 60)

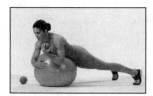

Off-the-Ball Curls (page 63)

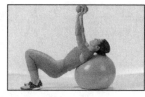

Chest-Press Incline (page 64)

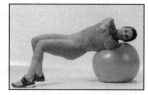

Arm-Swing Rolls (page 65)

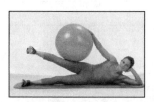

Thigh Buster (page 66)

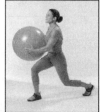

Atlas Lunge (page 68)

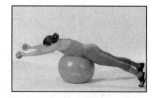

Flying Carpet (page 69)

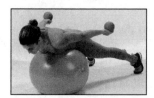

Triceps Extension (page 70)

Day 37

The old you, the one who hated exercise, is fading. The new you, the one open to new possibilities, is blooming.

Check off your pyramid servings:

Wholegrain
  breads/starches ❏ ❏ ❏ ❏ ❏ ❏ ❏ ❏ ❏ ❏   _____ servings

Vegetables ❏ ❏ ❏ ❏   _____ servings

Fruits ❏ ❏ ❏ ❏   _____ servings

Calcium-rich foods ❏ ❏ ❏   _____ servings

Protein-rich foods ❏ ❏ ❏ ❏ ❏ ❏ ❏   _____ servings

Healthful fats ❏ ❏ ❏ ❏ ❏   _____ servings

Today I ate these smarter protein, carbohydrate, fluid, and fat choices:

_____

_____

_____

_____

_____

_____

Today I ate these troublesome protein, carbohydrate, fluid, and fat choices:

_____

_____

_____

_____

_____

Tomorrow I will try to eat smarter by:

_____

_____

_____

_____

_____

_____

Today I ate this for dessert (name and amount):

_____

_____

_____

_____

_____

_____

Day 37 Tip: *Listen to your favorite music when you exercise. It will help you pick up the pace.*

Day 37 Workout: *Walk for 35 minutes today. Warm up for 5 minutes with slower walking and then pump your arms as you pick up the pace. Walk at a fast clip for 5 minutes and then slow down to your normal pace for 2 minutes. Continue alternating between 5 minutes of faster walking and 2 minutes of slower walking for the next 25 minutes. Cool down with 5 minutes at an easy pace.*

Day 38

See your anger, stress, and frustration as no more than a hormonal surge without an outlet. Every time you feel negative emotions, go for a brisk walk. You'll quickly leave negativity behind.

Check off your pyramid servings:

Wholegrain
  breads/starches ❑ ❑ ❑ ❑ ❑ ❑ ❑ ❑ ❑ ❑ _____ servings

Vegetables ❑ ❑ ❑ ❑ _____ servings

Fruits ❑ ❑ ❑ ❑ _____ servings

Calcium-rich foods ❑ ❑ ❑ _____ servings

Protein-rich foods ❑ ❑ ❑ ❑ ❑ ❑ ❑ _____ servings

Healthful fats ❑ ❑ ❑ ❑ ❑ _____ servings

Today I ate these smarter protein, carbohydrate, fluid, and fat choices:

_____

_____

_____

_____

_____

_____

Today I ate these troublesome protein, carbohydrate, fluid, and fat choices:

_____

_____

_____

_____

_____

_____

Tomorrow I will try to eat smarter by:

_____

_____

_____

_____

_____

Today I ate this for dessert (name and amount):

_____

_____

_____

_____

_____

Day 38 Tip: *Are your clothes hanging on you? That's because your body shape has changed! Celebrate by purchasing a new outfit. Your new clothes will flatter your figure and renew your motivation to stick with your fitness program.*

Day 38 Workout:

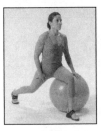

Seated Leg Stretch
(page 17)

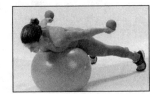

Triceps Extension
(page 70)

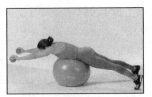

Flying Carpet
(page 69)

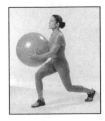

Atlas Lunge (page 68)

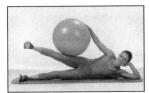

Thigh Buster (page 66)

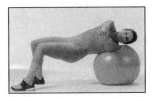

Arm-Swing Rolls
(page 65)

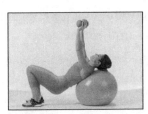

Chest-Press Incline
(page 64)

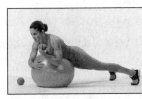

Off-the-Ball Curls
(page 63)

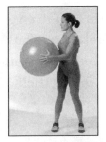

Standing Torso Twist
(page 60)

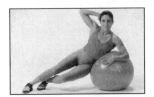

Side-Ups (page 59)

Day 39

Your exercise partner may be no farther away than the house next door. Ask one of your neighbors to join you for a walk.

Check off your pyramid servings:

Wholegrain
   breads/starches ❏ ❏ ❏ ❏ ❏ ❏ ❏ ❏ ❏ ❏   _____ servings

Vegetables ❏ ❏ ❏ ❏   _____ servings

Fruits ❏ ❏ ❏ ❏   _____ servings

Calcium-rich foods ❏ ❏ ❏   _____ servings

Protein-rich foods ❏ ❏ ❏ ❏ ❏ ❏ ❏   _____ servings

Healthful fats ❏ ❏ ❏ ❏ ❏   _____ servings

Today I ate these smarter protein, carbohydrate, fluid, and fat choices:

_____

_____

_____

_____

_____

_____

Today I ate these troublesome protein, carbohydrate, fluid, and fat choices:

_____

_____

_____

_____

_____

Tomorrow I will try to eat smarter by:

_____

_____

_____

_____

_____

_____

Today I ate this for dessert (name and amount):

_____

_____

_____

_____

_____

_____

Day 39 Tip: *To gauge your progress, focus on how your clothes fit and the positive comments you receive from others. Forget the numbers on the scale. A woman's weight can change dramatically from day to day, just from water retention. Because muscle weighs more than fat, the number on the scale may not even provide a true indication of your fitness.*

Day 39 Workout: *Walk for 35 minutes today. Warm up for 5 minutes with slower walking and then pump your arms as you pick up the pace. Walk at a fast clip for 5 minutes and then slow down to your normal pace for 2 minutes. Continue alternating between 5 minutes of faster walking and 2 minutes of slower walking for the next 25 minutes. Cool down with 5 minutes at an easy pace.*

Day 40

On the days when you manage to complete your workout despite hundreds of excuses not to, you take a huge step in your evolution toward a fitter you.

Check off your pyramid servings:

Wholegrain
  breads/starches ❏ ❏ ❏ ❏ ❏ ❏ ❏ ❏ ❏ ❏   _____ *servings*

Vegetables ❏ ❏ ❏ ❏   _____ *servings*

Fruits ❏ ❏ ❏ ❏   _____ *servings*

Calcium-rich foods ❏ ❏ ❏   _____ *servings*

Protein-rich foods ❏ ❏ ❏ ❏ ❏ ❏ ❏   _____ *servings*

Healthful fats ❏ ❏ ❏ ❏ ❏   _____ *servings*

Today I ate these smarter protein, carbohydrate, fluid, and fat choices:

_____

_____

_____

_____

_____

Today I ate these troublesome protein, carbohydrate, fluid, and fat choices:

_____

_____

_____

_____

_____

Tomorrow I will try to eat smarter by:

_____

_____

_____

_____

_____

Today I ate this for dessert (name and amount):

_____

_____

_____

_____

_____

Day 40 Tip: *Purchase some healthful cookbooks or sign up for a subscription to a cooking magazine. Sometimes eating healthier is simply a matter of mastering the tools of the trade.*

Day 40 Workout:

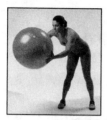

Around the World
(page 15)

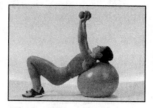

Chest-Press Incline
(page 64)

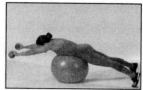

Flying Carpet
(page 69)

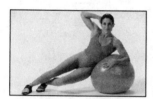

Side-Ups (page 59)

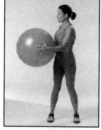

Standing Torso Twist
(page 60)

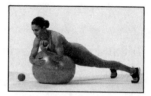

Off-the-Ball Curls
(page 63)

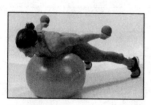

Triceps Extension
(page 70)

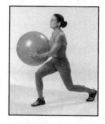

Atlas Lunge (page 68)

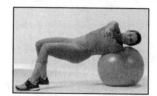

Arm-Swing Rolls
(page 65)

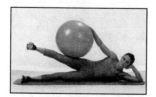

Thigh Buster (page 66)

Day 41

Do it for you, for your health, for your well-being, for your happiness. In the end, you're the one who must stick with the program.

Check off your pyramid servings:

Wholegrain breads/starches ❑ ❑ ❑ ❑ ❑ ❑ ❑ ❑ ❑ ❑	_____	servings
Vegetables ❑ ❑ ❑ ❑	_____	servings
Fruits ❑ ❑ ❑ ❑	_____	servings
Calcium-rich foods ❑ ❑ ❑	_____	servings
Protein-rich foods ❑ ❑ ❑ ❑ ❑ ❑ ❑	_____	servings
Healthful fats ❑ ❑ ❑ ❑ ❑	_____	servings

Today I ate these smarter protein, carbohydrate, fluid, and fat choices:

_____

_____

_____

_____

_____

_____

Today I ate these troublesome protein, carbohydrate, fluid, and fat choices:

_____

_____

_____

_____

_____

_____

Tomorrow I will try to eat smarter by:

_____

_____

_____

_____

_____

Today I ate this for dessert (name and amount):

_____

_____

_____

_____

_____

Day 41 Tip: *You're almost there! To encourage yourself to stick with your new healthy habits beyond six weeks, take yourself shopping. Buy a new exercise outfit. There's nothing like a small financial investment to encourage yourself to stick to a fitness investment.*

Day 41 Workout: *Walk for 35 minutes today. Warm up for 5 minutes with slower walking and then pump your arms as you pick up the pace. Walk at a fast clip for 5 minutes and then slow down to your normal pace for 2 minutes. Continue alternating between 5 minutes of faster walking and 2 minutes of slower walking for the next 25 minutes. Cool down with 5 minutes at an easy pace.*

Day 42

Congratulations! You completed the program. But don't stop here. Your life awaits you!

Check off your pyramid servings:

Wholegrain
  breads/starches ❑ ❑ ❑ ❑ ❑ ❑ ❑ ❑ ❑ ❑   _____ servings

Vegetables ❑ ❑ ❑ ❑   _____ servings

Fruits ❑ ❑ ❑ ❑   _____ servings

Calcium-rich foods ❑ ❑ ❑   _____ servings

Protein-rich foods ❑ ❑ ❑ ❑ ❑ ❑ ❑   _____ servings

Healthful fats ❑ ❑ ❑ ❑ ❑   _____ servings

Today I ate these smarter protein, carbohydrate, fluid, and fat choices:

_____

_____

_____

_____

_____

_____

Today I ate these troublesome protein, carbohydrate, fluid, and fat choices:

_____

_____

_____

_____

_____

Tomorrow I will try to eat smarter by:

_____

_____

_____

_____

Today I ate this for dessert (name and amount):

_____

_____

_____

_____

Day 42 Tip: *You completed the six-week body makeover, but this isn't the end for you. Because today is your day off, take some time to plan your fitness future. Go back to chapter 5 and recalculate your calories. Perhaps it's time to switch to a new weight-loss pyramid. Also, think about ways you can stick with your fitness habits for life. Perhaps you can do your ball workout with a friend. You might split up your walking time, doing part in the morning, part at lunch, and part after work. Commit yourself to a lifetime of fitness and healthy eating. List as many ways that you can think of to make your goal come true.*

My fitness and eating goals:

_____

_____

_____

_____

*Signature*_____

Day 42 Workout: *Today is your day off. Celebrate the new you!*

PART THREE

your personal approach

8

six weeks and beyond

Customizing your ball routine to your personal interests and needs to help you stick with the program for life

When I first learned how to exercise with a fitness ball, I relied on my physical therapist to tell me what moves to do and in what order to do them.

I did the workouts that he suggested, and I did them religiously. However, it wasn't until I went in one day and told Bill, "I want to show you something" that I knew this new ball concept was going to stick with me for life. While Bill watched, I perched myself on the ball, balancing on my shins with my body in an upright position like an elephant at a circus. Then I slowly lowered my upper body to the floor, all the while keeping my shins balanced on the ball.

"What do you think?" I asked him.

"You've just invented your very own ball exercise," he said. "You've targeted your whole core and your shoulder muscles." I was getting praise from a real pro, and I felt ecstatic.

As time went by, I relied on Bill less and less to tell me how to use the exercise ball. I began making up more and more of my own moves and designing my own routines. I now had the freedom to target the muscle groups I felt needed the most work on a particular day and to design workouts that I looked forward to and that fit into my schedule.

I'd like you to experience that freedom.

During the first six weeks of your program, I gave you a detailed prescription. I showed you specific exercises to do and told you what order to do them in. Many women just starting a new fitness program tell me that they want that kind of detail. They tell me that they don't want to make decisions. They just want to know what to do and when to do it.

As time goes on, though, most women opt for more freedom. That's what this chapter is all about. It will give you the tools you need to design a ball workout that fits into your schedule, a ball workout that works for you, a ball workout that blends perfectly into your life.

If you're not yet ready for this kind of freedom, don't worry. You don't *have* to start designing your own workouts. As you keep exercising beyond six weeks, you can simply continue to cycle through the three routines I suggested in chapter 2. You can also try the advanced routine in chapter 3.

If you are ready for more freedom, read on. Your options truly are endless.

Your Body, Your Ball

To understand how to customize ball workouts to your personal needs, you first must understand some basic physiology. Don't worry: This isn't going to be like high school physics or biology class.

To firm your body symmetrically, you need to work all the major muscle groups: the abs, back, legs, shoulders, biceps, triceps, and chest. Some women try to cheat by only working the area of their body that annoys them the most, usually their abs or rear end. This approach won't build lean muscle throughout your body. You want lean muscle to boost your metabolic rate and let you burn calories while you sleep. You can only do that by working your entire body.

Also, selecting only certain muscle groups to work on may create muscle imbalances that can lead to discomfort or even injury. For example, working your abs but not your back could lead to back pain.

So when designing your routines, include at least one exercise from each of the following ten muscle groups:

- Abs
- Back (upper)
- Back (lower)
- Biceps (upper arms)
- Chest
- Core
- Legs (butt and calves)
- Legs (thighs)
- Shoulders
- Triceps (upper arms)

That doesn't mean you can't put a little extra emphasis on body parts that may need it, such as your thighs, but it does mean you can't leave any muscle group out simply because you don't feel the need to tone it.

Mixing and matching the exercises in this book won't take a degree in physiology. All of the suggested exercises in chapters 2, 3, and 9 include labels that say what muscle group they target. You can also use the chart in chapter 3 on page 74 for quick reference.

A Routine Exercise

Over time, I hope you rely less and less on the workouts in this book and more and more on your inner coach, the one that intuitively knows what your body needs. Relying on your inner coach rather than

Move This Way

When designing your own moves, always keep safety in mind. Here are some tips:

Make sure you have enough space. When pairing exercises together, first look around and mentally see yourself doing the exercise. Will you bang into the coffee table? Will you slip on a dog toy? Make sure you have enough space to do the whole combination safely.

Stay in a neutral position. Keep your head centered above your shoulders (not jutting forward or tipped upward) and your spine long. Periodically remind yourself of this position by standing against a wall and lining your head, shoulders, upper back, and buttocks against the wall.

Never hyperextend. When making up new moves, remember not to arch your back or neck above the plane of your torso. This will help keep you from straining your spine, particularly if you already have a herniated disc or other degenerative spinal condition.

Be careful when lifting and twisting. If you have weak back muscles, extending them and twisting them at the same time may be too hard for you. You may pull a muscle a little too hard and create postexercise soreness.

Listen to your body. No exercise should hurt, particularly at a joint. You should feel the move in the center of your muscles, not at the ends where they attach to the joints. If you feel pain, don't do the move. At the end of your workout, you want your muscles to feel fatigued, not beat up.

on standard routine will allow you to tone your body more effectively, increase your enjoyment and motivation, and allow you to more easily overcome time constraints and other barriers to exercise.

The following tips will help you add variety and customize your routine to your personal needs. You don't need to cram all of my suggestions into your next workout. Rather, read through these tips and note the ones that seem most interesting to you right now. In a month or so, read through them again and choose others to further customize your workout.

Keep It Fresh   Try to change your program at least once a week. Adding a new exercise, tweaking an old one, or switching the order of the same exercises will keep your program fresh and your motivation strong. You might design one workout with moves from chapter 2, working your muscle groups in alphabetical order from your abs to triceps. You might design another by doing those very same moves in reverse alphabetical order or by working your muscles in order from head to toe, starting with your chest and upper back, then moving to your arms, your abs, core, lower back, and so on. You also might try one new move during each routine, perhaps an advanced move from chapter 3.

Make the Best of Your "Rest" Time   Try to make your ball workout somewhat aerobic by alternating your ball exercises with heart-pumping moves such as jumping jacks, jogging in place, shadow boxing, and skipping. Also, go back to the ball balances you learned in chapter 1. Or, simply bounce on top of your ball. It may seem like more fun than work, but bouncing will work your calves, core, and quadriceps and also improve your balance. Always try to put your rest break between moves to good, fun use.

If you're pressed for time, you might perform short chores during your rest break. Stir the soup that's simmering on the stove, gather shoes and put them in the closet, or straighten that unruly pile of magazines on the coffee table.

Use Your Imagination   Experiment with new exercises from your own personal repertoire. To figure out what muscles your new exercises work on, listen to your body as you work out. You'll be able to feel the muscles move.

To get started, alter the exercises you learned in chapters 2 and 3. You might try the Butt Lift with bent knees or do the Chest-Press Incline while in a modified bridge with your feet on the ball and shoulders on the mat. You might try the Big Squeeze with extended legs. Or how about incorporating the ball into other exercise moves you already know—you might use it as a prop for the Triangle in Yoga or the V-sit in Pilates. Even holding the ball over your head as you bend forward into a forward bend with legs either close together or wide apart will work the backs of your thighs.

Experiment. Have fun. Turn off your inner critic. Turn on your inner coach. That's what this program is all about.

Change Up the Sequence   If you're short on time, try eliminating rest breaks. Rather than completing one set of an exercise, resting, and then completing a second set of the same exercise, run through your program doing just one set of each exercise, and then run through the program again to do the second set of each.

You can also try working opposing muscle groups. When you contract your chest muscles, the muscles in your upper back will stretch. When you contract your biceps, the triceps along the backs of your upper arms will stretch. Working opposing groups back to back allows you to move through your routine without resting. To see how this works, try doing one exercise for your biceps, then one for your triceps. Go back to biceps and repeat. You can also alternate upper body moves with lower body moves.

Finally, try doing two to three different exercises for each muscle group without a break. Let's say you are starting with your abs. You'd do the regular crunch, the reverse crunch, and then the side crunch all in a row without a rest break.

Blast Your Trouble Spots   I know I told you to work your body in a balanced manner. It's absolutely a bad idea to work just a couple of muscle groups in isolation and ignore the rest of your body. However, it is perfectly safe to work some muscle groups a little bit *harder* than the rest of your body.

I like to pick a trouble spot to blast during each of my ball workouts. One day I might pick core exercises. Another day it might be my legs or abs. Between every single exercise, I toss in a move targeting that muscle group. If I'm blasting my abs, I'll do a chest press and then an abdominal crunch, a biceps curl and then a reverse crunch, a triceps extension and then an obliques crunch, and so on. By the end of the workout, my abs are crying for a rest.

Combine Similar Moves   If your routine starts to feel *too* routine, try to make it a little more exciting by flowing from one exercise into another. Start by grouping exercises that require the same basic ball position, maybe in a bridge or reverse bridge. Then flow from one exercise directly into another without a break. You might group Push-Ups with Knee Fold-Ups, Chest Flies with Drop Squats, X Marks the Spot with Stomach Back Flies. You also might try doing your workout without a preconceived plan. Start in the bridge position and see how many exercises you can do from it. Then lie prone on the ball and see how many exercises you can do. You get the picture.

Just Balance   I've started a little contest with myself to see how long I can balance on my ball in various positions. One day I'll sit on the ball with my feet in the air and watch the clock as I shimmy from side to side and attempt to stay in place without putting my feet down. Another day I'll try balancing from a kneeling position or even a flying-wonder-woman position with my tummy on the ball.

With each attempt, I try to beat my previous time. This little contest helps me fit in a mini workout without even noticing that I've worked out.

Sit on It   Perch yourself on the ball while you perform other tasks. That way, you'll work your core and legs whenever you get the chance. Occasionally, I like to use my ball as a chair at my computer workstation. As I answer e-mail, I subconsciously bounce and move around on the ball. In addition to working my muscles, it also helps keep me alert.

Name Your Moves   I'm not attached to the names I've given the exercises in this book. If you want to name them after your dog, your kids, or anything else that strikes your fancy, go right ahead. Giving the moves customized names makes it more likely that you will remember them.

Break It Up   If you're as busy as I am, you may have trouble finding 30 spare minutes in the day. That's fine. It doesn't mean you can't work out. Just break up the routine a little. For example, sometimes I find that I have 10 minutes before I must leave to pick up my daughter from swim practice. I'll fit in some moves during that 10 minutes, go pick up Natalie, and then do some more when I return. If you try this method, group like muscles together, such as your chest and back, your arms and shoulders, and so on. That will help you remember where you left off.

9

a ball for
every body

Play tennis? Need an exercise partner? Short on time? Find a
customized ball routine that's exactly right for you!

I love fitness balls so much that I can't stop gushing about all of their
wonders.

Perhaps their greatest strength lies in their universality. The ball
program benefits all women of all ages and all interests.

If you play sports, the core strength you gain from your ball program will help you run faster and jump higher. It will put more oomph
in your tennis stroke or golf swing. The ball program is so effective and
modifiable that you can use it to train for just about every fitness pursuit you can think of.

If you're not athletic but simply want to look and feel your best,
you can use the customized ball program to help you stand taller, tone
away flab, and blast away trouble spots.

If you've always wanted to get fit but had trouble scheduling an exercise program because of family, work, or social demands, you can
use the ball program to do two things at once. The workout is so efficient that you can fit in a great routine in just 15 minutes. It's so much
fun that you can do it with family members or friends.

No matter your goals, interests, or time constraints, you can create a ball routine that fits perfectly into your life and that harmonizes with your interests and goals. In the following pages, you'll find everything you need to customize your ball routine to your individual goals and lifestyle.

Customized Routines for Women Short on Time

All of us have days when a full 30- to 45-minute workout is simply impossible.

That's fine. Let's talk about just 15 minutes.

Most of us can find 15 minutes of downtime in a day. Think of the 15 minutes you wait for chicken to defrost in the microwave or for a big pot of water to boil. How about the 15 minutes your teenager monopolizes the bathroom or telephone when you need it? Or maybe the 15 minutes of brain rebellion between tasks at work when you *should* be busy but can't motivate yourself to pick up that next piece of paper?

These are all perfect times to fit in a workout.

You can condense the typical 30-minute ball workout into 15 minutes or less simply by eliminating your rest breaks between sets.

When I'm short on time, I alternate between two similar moves that work different body parts. I might do a series of Classic Crunches and then pick up the heavy balls that I've stashed nearby and roll right into a series of Chest-Press Inclines. After one set of Chest-Press Inclines, I do more Classic Crunches. As I crunch, my chest muscles get the chance to recover. As I do my chest exercise, my abs recover. By alternating, I can keep moving without taking a break.

Try to combine exercises that require the same position on the ball. That way, you eliminate the few seconds it takes to switch from a prone position to a bridge, for example.

Great combinations that I've tried include:

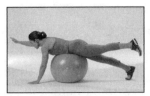 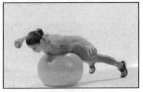

X Marks the Spot (page 48) with Stomach Back Flies (page 49)

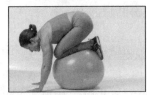 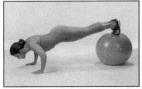

Push-Offs (page 45) with Push-Ups (page 38)

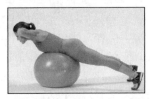 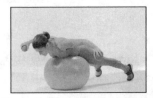

Knee Fold-Ups (page 40) with Push-Ups (page 38)

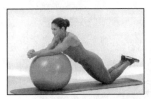 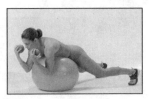

Upper Torso Lift (page 33) with Stomach Back Flies (page 49)

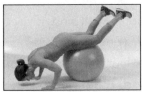 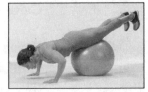

Kneeling Layouts (page 53) with Preacher Ball Curls (page 36)

Just remember that you are saving time by eliminating the rest break between sets, not by doing your reps faster. Continue to move through the exercises in a slow and controlled fashion.

To save even more time, try combining two exercises into one, as in the following example.

DROP SQUAT SHOULDER PRESS

For the Drop Squat Shoulder Press, I combine the Chest Flies from chapter 2 with a Drop Squat to work my upper body and lower body in just one exercise.

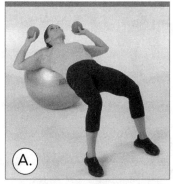

A. Lie in a bridge position with your shoulders on the ball, your knees bent, and your feet flat on the floor. Grasp a pair of heavy balls in each hand. Hold them with your elbows bent out to the sides and the balls just above your collarbones.

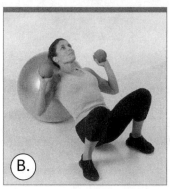

B. Inhale as you squat down by bringing your buttocks closer to the floor and bending your knees even more. Roll your back along the ball as you do this.

C. Exhale as you press the heavy balls up, extending your arms overhead. Lower your arms and push yourself back into a bridge position. Repeat 10 to 15 times.

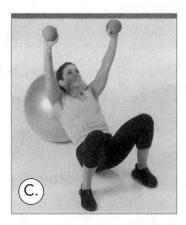

You can combine Bridge-Back Curls and other upper body moves with the Drop Squat. You might also try doing Side-Ups while lifting your extended top leg to work your outer thigh. Or, when doing Triceps Extensions, lift one leg up and squeeze your buttocks for half of your reps. Then lift the other leg and work your buns as you work your upper arms.

Customized Routines for Spots That Need Extra Attention

I know few women who can't point to an area somewhere on their body that they'd like to tone up just a tad more. These trouble spots include the hips, thighs, buttocks, abs, or triceps—the typical fat depots that we all inherited from our cave-dwelling ancestors.

The ball routines in chapters 2 and 3 will help you tone those trouble spots as well as boost your metabolism by building muscle all over your body. To shape up those same trouble spots quickly, try doing some giant sets during your routines.

A giant set includes two or more exercises for the same muscle group. You complete the exercises in sequence (slow and controlled) without a rest break and then run through another set or two, completely fatiguing every area of that muscle group. You'll be shaking by the time your done!

The following are some great giant sets to try for different trouble spots.

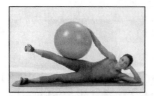
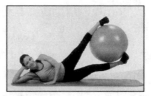

For your thighs, try Thigh Buster (page 66) with Scissors Lift (page 86)

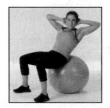
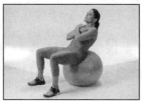
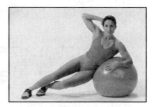

For your tummy, try the Oblique Twist (page 78),
Classic Crunches (page 31), and Side-Ups (page 59)

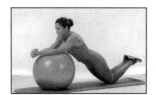
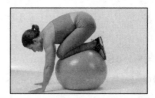

For your tummy, try Kneeling Layouts (page 53) with
Knee Fold-Ups (page 40)

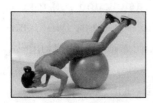
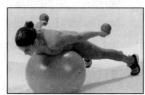
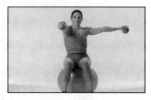

For your upper arms, try Push-Offs (page 45) with Triceps Extensions
(page 70) and Right-Angle Lateral Lifts (page 56)

If your thighs are your trouble spot, try the Thigh Buster with the
Scissors Lift from above and finish them off with the Big and Little
Squeeze shown on the following page.

THE BIG AND LITTLE SQUEEZES

(A.) For the Big Squeeze, lie on the mat with your legs bent and the ball between your knees. Place your hands at your sides. While squeezing your inner thighs against the ball, lift the ball about a foot from the mat as you slightly lift your shoulders. Be sure to work both your abs and your inner thighs. Keep your neck relaxed rather than straining it forward. Hold the position for 3 to 5 seconds, release, and repeat. You should feel this in your inner thighs, buttocks, and lower abs.

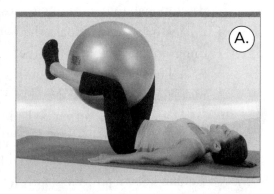

(B.) For the Little Squeeze, lie prone with your tummy and chest on the fitness ball and the balls of your feet against the mat. Place a small heavy ball in the bend behind one of your knees and then lift your calf to hold it in place. Without arching your back, pull, or bring, your calf toward your thigh, squeezing the ball for 3 to 5 seconds. Relax and repeat before switching legs. You should feel this in your buttocks and hamstrings.

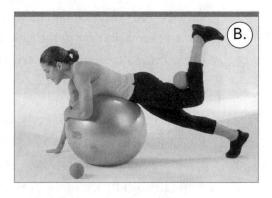

Customized Routines for Family and Friends

Including your children, husband, or friends in your ball workouts will boost your motivation as well as help you multitask.

I like to work out with my friend Kris or with my teenage daughter, Natalie. With Kris, I'll do a set of my exercises on the ball and then pass the ball to her during my rest break. She does her set then passes it back to me. As we pass the ball back and forth, we chat about anything and everything, and before we know it, we've completely fatigued our bodies. We encourage each other to do more reps, and this makes each of us work harder. We laugh and generally have a ball.

With Natalie, I often do ball stretches. All of the stretches in chapter 1—Around the World, Low Body Stretch, Buddha, and the Seated Leg Stretch—are safe for children. To do the Low Body Stretch, Natalie takes a position on my left. I roll the ball in a semicircle around my body from my right side to my left. When I've reached the full stretch on the left, Natalie takes the ball on her right, rolls it to her left, and then rolls it back to the right to me. We continue to pass the rolling ball off to each other as we stretch and have a mother-daughter chat.

We also do the Buddha Stretch together. We both assume the Buddha pose, with Natalie on one side of the ball and me on the other. Or we may alternate doing Around the World. First I do a cycle, then I pass the ball to her so she can do a cycle and send it back to me.

In addition to stretching with your children, you can also do a mini workout with them if they are old enough. Just make sure they use the right size ball for their height (see chart on page 4 in chapter 1). Two great exercises for kids include X Marks the Spot for coordination and Push-Offs for fun.

Two other fun exercises to do with your kids are Ball Fighting and Ball Tapping. You'll find yourself laughing as you work your abs, shoulders, upper back, and legs.

BALL FIGHTING

A. Stand facing your child with the ball between you. You should each grasp the ball at about chest level. (If your child is much shorter than you, you might go on your knees while your child stands.)

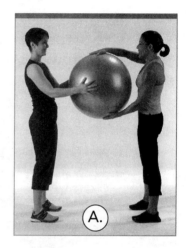

B. "Fight" with your child over the ball, rotating it from side to side as you wrangle for 15 seconds. Rest and repeat. Start out gently and increase the vigor of your rotation gradually. Be careful not to wrest the ball out of your child's hands.

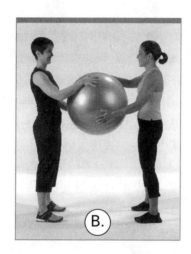

BALL TAPPING

A. Stand holding the ball at chest level with your arms extended and a slight bend at the elbows. (If your child is much shorter than you, go on your knees while your child stands.)

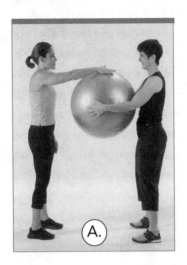

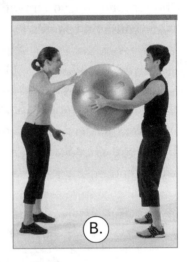

B. Ask your child to try to knock the ball out of your hands by tapping different parts of it from different directions. If you want to increase the difficulty (and fun) of the exercise, close your eyes as your child taps the ball. After 15 seconds, switch positions and let your child hold the ball as you tap.

Customized Routines for Golfers

If you only golf once a week or so, you know only too well that your muscles are never fully in shape for a day on the links. End result: You ache after every single outing.

This is where the ball program can help you. You can strengthen the shoulder, back, abdominal, and leg muscles you need for golf so that you're ready for those occasional days on the course. Even if you play often, by strengthening your core you can put more oomph in your swing and maintain your energy and concentration for all eighteen holes.

The following exercises will help you improve your game by strengthening the muscles you use to twist your body, swing your clubs, bend down to pick up the ball or the club that you threw, and walk the course. (No golf carts, please!)

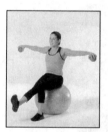

Lateral Lifts (page 89)

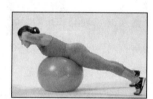

Upper Torso Lift (page 33)

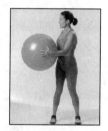

Standing Torso Twist (page 60)

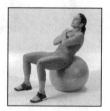

Classic Crunches (page 31)

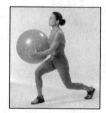

Atlas Lunge (page 68)

CHIP SHOT

The Chip Shot, one of the most effective fitness ball exercises for golf, helps train your body to twist. It works numerous large and small muscles in your torso, abdomen, and lower back.

A. Stand with your feet in your golf stance. Hug a heavy ball to your chest with both hands. Rotate your torso to the right while keeping your hips stationary and pointing forward.

B. Quickly rotate your torso to the left and continue to rotate back and forth from right to left quickly for 15 times on each side. Rest and repeat.

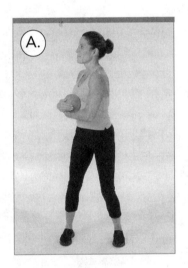
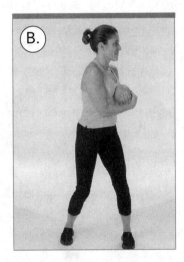

Customized Routines for Swimmers

Swimming uses just about every muscle in your body. Your upper body muscles pull your arms through the water, your core keeps you afloat, and your lower body pushes off the swimming pool wall and propels you through the water.

Your ball program will strengthen all of those muscles, particularly your core, and will help keep your hips, chest, and shoulders properly positioned in the water. To best prepare your body for swimming, use a lighter heavy ball and increase your number of repetitions to 30 during each exercise. This increase will help build the kind of muscular endurance you need in the pool.

Exercises to help you become a better swimmer include:

Triceps Extensions (page 70) Triceps Extensions mimic the end of your arm stroke as you extend your arm out of the water during freestyle. In the pool, you extend each arm as many as 24 times every 25 meters, so do as many repetitions as you can of this exercise.

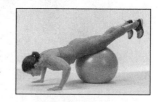

Push-Ups (page 38) Push-Ups work your chest and biceps, the muscles that help pull your arms under your body and through the water during freestyle.

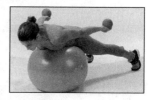

Stomach Back Flies (page 49) Swimmers often develop a strength imbalance between the internal rotators in front of their shoulders and the external rotators behind them. Weak externals and strong internals will pull the shoulders forward. This is why some swimmers have such poor posture. This exercise strengthens the external rotators and helps pull your shoulders back and open your chest.

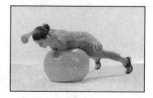

DOUBLE PUSH-OFFS

Try Double Push-Offs to help you develop more strength as you push yourself off the wall during every flip turn. It works your biceps, chest, back, and legs. During a typical swim workout, you might push off the wall 60 times, so this exercise will really help.

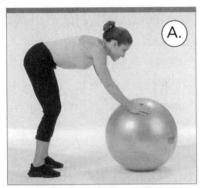

A. Stand with the ball 2 feet or so in front of your feet. Bend forward and place your hands on the ball.

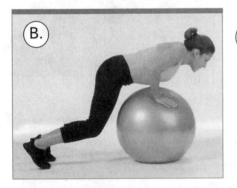

B. Bend your arms and lower yourself onto the ball as if you were lowering into a push-up on the ball.

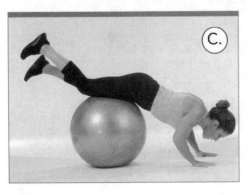

C. Slide your arms and then your torso along the ball, eventually pushing off from your feet as you roll forward. Land with your palms on the floor and your feet in the air. You should look as if you were diving into a swimming pool. When your palms reach the floor, bend your elbows and lower your face toward the floor. Then push off through your palms, bringing your feet back to the floor as your torso rolls the ball back. Rise to the starting position and repeat 10 to 12 times.

Customized Routines for Snow Sports

Few people ski or snowboard every day or even every week. Even if you perform other strenuous exercises on a regular basis, you won't mimic the motions you go through on the slopes. That means you'll tire easily and feel extremely sore the day after every skiing or snowboarding excursion, unless you put the ball to work for you.

The following exercises will help tone important muscles in your legs, back, and abdomen.

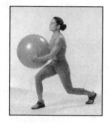

Atlas Lunge
(page 68)

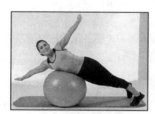

Torso Lift and Twist
(page 82)

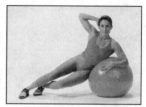

Side-Ups
(page 59)

WALL SQUATS

The Wall Squat does the best job of mimicking your body position on the slopes. It helps build up the quad strength you need to make numerous runs without fatigue.

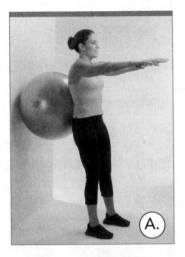

A. Position a fitness ball between your lower back and the wall. Lean into the ball and take one step away from the wall with both feet.

B. Press back into the ball as you squat down, bringing your buttocks closer to the floor. Only bend your knees as far as it feels comfortable, up to 90 degrees. Press through your feet to rise to the starting position. Repeat 10 to 15 times. Then lower and hold for 30 seconds, eventually working up to a 90-second hold. To make the move more challenging, place a heavy ball between your knees and press your thighs inward during the wall squat.

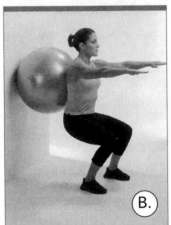

Customized Routines for Tennis Players

Like swimmers, tennis players often develop a muscle imbalance between their internal and external rotators in their chest, shoulders, and upper back. Heavy hitting of the ball both on serve and returning strokes can combine with this muscle imbalance to lead to rotator cuff tears, shoulder bursitis, and other common tennis injuries.

The following exercises will help strengthen the muscles you need to hold up your racket, whack the tennis ball, and sprint from one end of the court to the other.

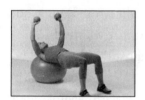

Chest Flies
(page 52)

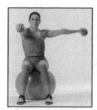

Right-Angle Lateral Lifts
(page 56)

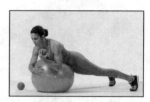

Off-the-Ball Curls
(page 63)

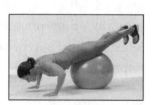

Push-Ups (page 38)

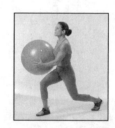

Atlas Lunge (page 68)

EXTERNAL ROTATION ON BALL

The External Rotation exercise will firm up your external rotators and help minimize that muscle imbalance to save your shoulders from injury.

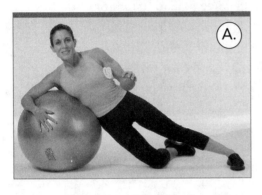

A. To open your shoulder joint, roll up a small hand towel and place it between your left arm and armpit. Lie on your right side on the fitness ball and hug the ball with your right arm. Bend your right leg and rest your right knee and shin against the floor. Extend your left leg. With your left arm bent in a 90-degree angle and the top of your left arm against your ribs, grasp a heavy ball (about 0.5 kg) in your left hand.

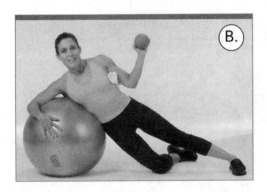

B. Rotate your left hand up, keeping your left elbow fixed against your ribs. Stop once your hand reaches the plane of your body. Repeat 10 to 12 times.

Customized Routines for Runners

Runners notoriously ignore their upper bodies when strength training (if they strength train at all). But runners need upper-body strength to pump their arms and hold their bodies upright as they run. Without upper-body strength, runners slump forward.

The ball program helps strengthen your upper body and will help you press your chest forward and pull your shoulders back as you run. When you're in this posture, you naturally increase your gait.

Do the Chest-Press Inclines and Arm-Swing Rolls in particular, because they also target the leg muscles. Also, do the Buddha Stretch regularly to stretch out your backside.

BUTT LIFT AND CURL

This exercise combination works just about every leg muscle involved in running. It will help you tackle hills with more ease, and you will have more endurance during a long run.

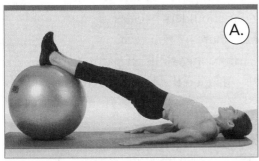

A. Lie with your back on the mat, your arms at your sides, and your heels on top of the fitness ball. Do butt lifts by pressing your hips up to form a straight line from your heels to your elbows. Repeat 10 times.

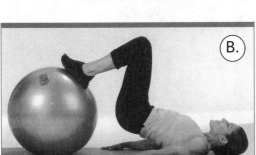

B. Now do hamstring curls, using your heels to pull the ball in toward your buttocks. Repeat 10 times.

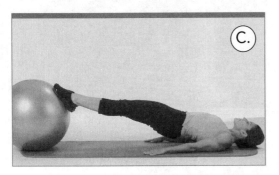

C. Walk the ball backward away from your buttocks as you straighten your legs. Balancing with only the tips of your toes against the ball, form a straight line from your toes to your shoulders. For the final set, do more butt lifts, pressing your hips toward the ceiling. Repeat 10 times. Great for your legs and butt!

PART FOUR

beautiful
for life

10

when life intervenes

How to follow your ball program and dessert diet at restaurants, at work, when traveling, and when under stress

Have you ever gone out to eat with friends only to realize 800 calories later, after a plate of nachos and two margaritas, that you've blown your diet?

Or maybe you blew it after flying from New York to San Francisco when you snacked on all those cheese fries, Cokes, and hot dogs during the layover in St. Louis. Or was it late last night, when you ate an entire pint of Ben and Jerry's standing before the refrigerator as you fretted over an argument with that certain someone?

No doubt about it, some situations tempt us to eat more than we should. Even when we're following a no-deprivation, eat-dessert-every-single-day diet, there are times when we really want to dig into troublesome food. Fortunately, you can get a handle on these situations. The most common triggers for overeating are eating out, stress, and travel. Let's take a look at ways to overcome each of these fitness-sabotaging situations.

Eat Less When Eating Out

Few people eat out without muttering, "I wish I hadn't eaten so much." Research clearly shows that most of us not only eat too much food but also eat too much of the wrong types of foods when we eat out.

You could opt to eat at home. But I know that's not realistic in these times when survey after survey shows that more people are eating out more often. Restaurant eating has become part of American culture. To stay nutritionally fit, you have no choice but to learn how to make better choices away from your own kitchen.

Here are some tips.

Plan on Portion Control   Most restaurants pack your plate with more than you normally eat. To keep yourself from overeating, you must have a plan. You might split your entrée with a friend, order two appetizers instead of a main course, or ask the wait staff to stick half of your meal into a take-out container *before* they bring it to your table. Ask for smaller portions or order a half portion if the restaurant offers it. Sometimes, simply *asking* the wait staff how large the portions are before you order can remind you of your diet and help you control your eating. My favorite ploy is to wear a tight outfit that gives me instant feedback when I overdo it.

Look Before You Order   Before you enter a restaurant, check out the menu on the door or front window and search for grilled fish, fresh vegetable side dishes or salads, and healthful vegetarian entrées. If you don't find those items, move on to another eatery with more healthful choices.

Get Table Service   Avoid buffet tables and cafeteria-style restaurants. Opt instead for a sit-down restaurant where you order from a menu. According to nutrition-anthropologists, we're genetically programmed to taste everything when we see lots of food. One study showed that people ate more dessert calories when they were offered cookies, cheesecake, pudding, and other choices than when they were offered only cheesecake.

This is perhaps another throwback to our cave-dwelling ancestors, who wouldn't have survived if they didn't eat all the nuts, berries, and wild animals in sight. It also may be part of the American psyche and the philosophy that we must get the most food for our money.

When you must eat at a buffet, allow yourself just one selection of a particular course. Have only one appetizer, one side dish, one main dish, one dessert item, and one beverage. You'll automatically eat less, and you will still feel satisfied.

Try a Natural Predinner Appetite Suppressant   Before eating out, slip in a quick, vigorous workout to keep your appetite under control. In one study, a group of cyclists pedaled vigorously on a stationary bike for 30 minutes, another group pedaled slowly, and a third didn't exercise at all. When offered food 15 minutes later, the fast-pedaling cyclists weren't hungry. They pushed the food away, while the slow cyclists and the nonexercisers dug in. An hour before your dinner reservation, go for a brisk walk or do your ball workout. Really pump your arms and move at a fast clip. When you get to the restaurant, you will love your blunt appetite.

Drink Water Before Dining   After you finish your prerestaurant workout, drink plenty of water. In one study, people who ran on a treadmill for 50 minutes in the morning and then drank some water ate fewer calories later in the day than people who drank either a sugar-sweetened or artificially-flavored (zero-calorie) beverage. Something about the sweet taste of even a diet drink primes the belly to crave more food, whereas plain old-fashioned water reduces hunger.

Eat Less on the Road

Sometimes I travel so much that I forget the town or time zone I'm in. But I never forget my arsenal of eating and fitness strategies to help me stay trim while on the road. No matter how busy you are—or how much you travel—the following self-tested tips will help you eat nutritious meals and keep off unwanted pounds.

Plan Ahead   Before you take a trip, find out what facilities are available at the hotel or nearby. Ask about the hotel's fitness room and about local health clubs and rates. Does the hotel have an in-house restaurant? If so, ask them to e-mail or fax the menu to you so that you know what type of fare to expect.

Some extended-stay hotels offer kitchenettes with a refrigerator, microwave, and stove. If you have this option, make good use of it. As soon as you get to your destination, stop at a grocery store and stock up on breakfast items like whole-grain cereals, fresh fruit, and lowfat milk or soy milk. This way you can bypass that morning restaurant meal of pastries and cheese omelets that usually add up to unwanted calories and fat.

Always Eat Breakfast   Your brain is counting on you for needed fuel and nutrients to launch your workday or vacation, so never skip breakfast, no matter how pressed you are for time.

An ideal start-your-day-right meal supplies a good source of protein, carbohydrate, vitamins, minerals, and fiber. You don't need to eat out to satisfy all of these requirements. Instead, have a bowl of raisin bran topped with milk (cow's milk or soy) and fresh berries that you have stored in your hotel room mini refrigerator.

Don't Overlook Dried Fruit   Dried fruit is great because it requires no refrigeration and is one of the easiest and fastest ways to sneak in produce on the road. You can pack dried fruits in your briefcase or stash them in the car. Most processing techniques used to dry fruits only remove moisture and small amounts of vitamin C. Minerals such as potassium, iron, calcium (dried figs are a great source), phytochemicals, and vitamins stay put.

Make the Most of Frozen Dinners   If you're staying in a hotel room with a mini kitchenette, look no further than the frozen dinner aisle at the nearby grocery store for a low-calorie, healthful dinner option. Nix any dessert that comes with the dinner. Instead, finish off your meal with fresh berries topped with a touch of light whipped cream or yogurt. Frozen, no-sugar-added fruit, such as blueberries, peaches, and strawberries, sweetened with a drizzle of honey also make an easy vitamin-packed dessert.

Choose frozen dinners with:

- 300 to 500 calories per package

- No more than 10 to 15 grams of total fat and 2 to 5 grams of saturated fat

- 5 or more grams of fiber

Make the Most of the Salad Bar   All of my dessert-diet plans include at least four servings of fruit and vegetables daily, making the salad bar in the restaurant or supermarket one of your best nutritional allies on the road. Select dark green lettuces, fresh cut-up vegetables, beans, and sprouts and top it all off with an oil-and-vinegar dressing or just plain vinegar. Finish off with some fruit topped with yogurt.

Take Your Sneakers Everywhere   You're more likely to stick with your walking plan—whether on the road or at home—if you have easy access to your shoes. A pair of sneakers allows you to take a stress-releasing walk in a nearby park whenever you can sneak out for a break. Pack them in your suitcase and take them with you wherever you go. You never know when you'll find time to take that walk.

The same goes for your fitness ball. One of the best things about fitness balls is that you can deflate them and put them in a suitcase. Because the heavy balls may weigh down your suitcase, invest in some rubber tubing sold at sporting goods stores under the brand names Theraband, Dynaband, and others. The tubing provides resistance as you tug against it. You can secure it under your feet, body, or even a heavy chair and do the same exercises you would do with the heavy balls.

Make Time for Fitness   If you intentionally schedule some sort of exercise into your day on the road, you're more likely to do it. Plan on doing your exercise earlier in the day rather than later. Commitments tend to stack up as the day moves on, and there may be no time later for your workout.

Stay Moving on Travel Day   When in transit, it can be difficult to fit in formal exercise like jogging or an aerobics class. You can still stay in motion by walking around the airport terminal while you wait for your flight. If you're driving, stop for stretching and walking breaks. This will keep you from feeling sluggish while you also burn some calories.

Eat Less When You're Under Stress

Food can act as powerful medicine in the brain and can have both good and bad effects on the body. When it is beneficial, food serves as a trigger that alters the chemicals responsible for putting us in a good mood and keeping us calm. When food is harmful, it triggers other brain chemicals that make us feel jumpy or anxious. This harmful effect fuels a chain reaction: We eat because we're stressed. Then the food we eat makes us even more anxious. We eat more food and become more anxious, and on and on.

You see where I'm going. The next time you find yourself shoving food in your mouth during a hectic workday or an emotional crisis, follow these tips.

Call a Friend Often, talking about your bad day or stressful situation can help you calm down before you turn to food or before you turn to *too much* food.

Write It Down Jot down your thoughts—what you wanted to say to your boss but didn't dare—or anything else that may help calm your nerves. Therapists often suggest keeping a journal during stressful times. Writing down your feelings can get them out before you stuff them inside you with food.

Hit the Road Going for a walk or some other form of exercise is often the best medicine for stress. Studies show that a single stint of exercise can dramatically lift your mood. Walking or other activity also gets you away from the problem and allows you to mull over the situation and give you perspective.

Find a Distraction Focusing on another task can keep you away from the cookie jar. Run an errand, re-pot that overgrown houseplant, or replace those worn laces on your walking shoes. Do anything that will take your mind off the stress and take you away from a food stimulus that may lead to an eating-out-of-stress episode.

Go Single If sometimes you do yield and eat, opt for a single-serve cup or bar and savor it slowly. Don't buy a carton of ice cream! With a single portion, you control the calories.

Sip or Dip That Chocolate When chocolate is your comfort food of choice, sip on hot chocolate made with fat-free milk. Dipping fresh fruit, such as strawberries or pineapple chunks, in sweetened cocoa powder is another satisfying and nutritious way to lift your mood.

Opt for Hard Candy If you tend to eat everything in the kitchen when under stress, turn to foods that take a long time to eat or chew.

Hard candies will give you the sweet taste you seek, all for a mere 25 to 30 calories. Each candy takes a long time to finish off, so even if you binge, the calories don't add up fast.

Other slow-to-eat foods include nuts in the shell, frozen juice bars, and taffy.

Satisfy Salt Cravings with Alternatives   Some folks get solace from salty snacks like chips and snack crackers by the handful. To save calories, opt for salted air-popped popcorn or try ready-to-eat breakfast cereal mixed with soy nuts and pumpkin seeds. Drizzle this mixture with soy sauce and bake it in the oven. Now you have a salty snack loaded with protein, vitamins, and minerals.

For a crunchy texture, try a whole-grain, high-fiber breakfast cereal such as Wheat Chex. The high fiber content will quickly fill you up and put a stop to your eating episode before you go too far.

Eat Less at Work

Many of us find reasons to nosh at work. Some women eat out of boredom or procrastination, using the old line, "I'll finish filing these papers after I finish snacking on this candy bar." Others eat out of guilt, especially when a co-worker brings in treats and pleads with everyone to eat one, or two, or three, or more.

Then there are the people who are chained to their desks all day, except for when they get up to walk to the cafeteria, vending machine, or hotdog cart for a little sustenance to get them through the next hour.

No matter what causes you to fall off your diet plan at work, here are some ways to jump back on the wagon.

Plan Ahead   Take your own food to work. Stock your desk with survival, in-case-of-emergency foods such as instant soup mix, high protein or high-fiber cereal bars, dried fruit, trail mix, whole-grain crackers, protein powder, and cartons of shelf-stable milk.

Eat Breakfast   Starting your day with breakfast helps prevent low blood sugar that can lower your willpower when someone drops a dozen cinnamon buns off at your office. An ideal start-your-day-right meal supplies a good source of protein, carbohydrate, vitamins, minerals, and fiber. This is why ready-to-eat breakfast cereal topped with milk (cow's milk or soy) and fresh berries or another fruit counts as an ideal breakfast. Here are some other fast and nutritious morning meals.

- Toasted whole-grain bread spread with peanut butter and topped with a sliced banana

- Blender drink of yogurt mixed with orange juice, a banana, and a squirt of honey (makes for great sipping on a morning commute)

- Leftover vegetarian pizza with a glass of milk

- Goat cheese spread over a whole-wheat tortilla topped with tomato slices

- Cold, leftover cooked rice topped with dried fruit, almonds, brown sugar, and milk

Bring a Lunch   If you work in an environment where few healthful choices exist, you need to bring your own food to work. If you rarely pack a lunch, start with just once a week, then keep adding a day until you brown-bag it every day. Start with fast, easy-to-pack items like precut carrot sticks or other raw vegetables. Cauliflower, broccoli, celery, and radishes provide nice, low-calorie munching food that may satisfy your urge to chew during a stressful work episode.

Toss in a small carton of nonfat yogurt or cottage cheese for protein, or stick some imitation crabmeat in a baggie. Other quick and easy protein sources include a premade bean salad from the grocery store, sliced turkey in a pita, a hardboiled egg or soy burger (one quick minute in the office microwave and its ready to enjoy). Finish off your lunch with a piece of fruit or a mixture of blueberries, raspberries, and blackberries.

Avoid Vending Machines   Eating breakfast and packing your own lunch should help you avoid foraging at the vending machine. If a worst-case scenario arises, look for healthful options such as fruit, whole-grain cereal bars, nut mixes, and even peanut butter and crackers.

Just Say No   Find other ways to occupy yourself when co-workers bring in food. Come up with creative excuses, such as, "I'll try it right after I wash my hands" or, "Oh darn, I just ate a doughnut, but I'm sure your ice cream birthday cake is really good."

11

motivated for life

Spice up your program with plenty of variety,
and you'll never fall off the ball

Early during a new fitness program, your motivation remains naturally high for a number of reasons. For one thing, you're seeing results quickly and consistently.

In the first few weeks, if you want to lose weight, you'll see results every time you step on the scale or slip on a pair of pants. If you want to gain strength, you notice results during every single workout.

At some point after six weeks, results begin to slow. Eventually, you will reach your goal weight. Eventually, you will tone your muscles as much as they can get toned. Eventually, you will build up your strength and balance to their max.

After you reach these goals, you come to a cooling-off period. If you do nothing to motivate yourself during this time, you run the risk of falling off the ball permanently. You must convince yourself that to keep off the weight and maintain your firm, toned, strong muscles, you must stay on the program for life.

Unlike fad, lose-weight-fast diets, *Bounce Your Body Beautiful* provides you with a lifetime fitness program. Think of the first six weeks as your jump-start to a life of healthy fitness and eating habits.

To stick with your new healthy habits for *that long,* you must make them as enticing and interesting as possible. Otherwise, you run the risk of neglecting the fitness ball and finally storing it in the closet with your ab rollers and other gym equipment. Taking a few crucial proactive steps now will help strengthen your resolve in the years to come and make sure you get on the ball and stay on it for life.

Here are the most effective ways to fan your motivation, now and forever.

Focus on How You Feel   Whenever I don't feel like getting out of bed to do my work out, I remind myself that I'll feel better physically and mentally once I get moving. I repeat that to myself over and over, like a silent mantra. I manage to drag myself out of bed every single time. At night when I have an end-of-the-day workout planned and my motivation is waning, I focus on how energized and strong I'll feel when my workout is over.

Embark on an Adventure   Your new eating habits will seem more enticing if you focus on the expanding world of healthful and body-slimming new foods and meals waiting for you to try. See yourself as an intrepid explorer, out to sample that vast variety of exotic foods at your grocery store and in restaurants.

When eating out, order the local specialty, trying healthful, lowfat foods that you've never eaten before, perhaps sushi, ostrich, elk, or emu. Subscribe to a cooking magazine and try one new recipe a week. Buy one new food at the grocery store each week, such as mango, kohlrabi, or jicama. Learn how to peel a pineapple or mango. Experiment with different varieties of fish. If you've always cooked flounder, try grilling salmon or tuna steaks. If you've always eaten tuna sandwiches, try salmon sandwiches.

You may not like every new healthful food you try, but I guarantee you'll like enough of them to make eating a new adventure.

Change Your Workout   Doing the same moves in the same order workout after workout allows you to check out mentally, and sooner or later you not only no longer look forward to your workouts but also fail to work your muscles to fatigue. Periodically changing your program will keep your body and mind constantly challenged.

When you notice your mind drifting during your workouts, you need to change your routine. Challenge yourself with more reps, sets, or harder moves from chapter 3. Do the same routine in reverse order. Try to add a personal touch to each exercise.

Also, one or two days a week give a new cardio activity a try. Instead of walking, go for a bike ride or hop in a pool and swim laps. If you belong to a health club, give an aerobics or kick-boxing class a whirl or try a recumbent stationary bike or elliptical walker.

Tell Yourself You'll Only Do 10 Minutes   If you find yourself dreading your normal half-hour workout, commit yourself to only 10 minutes. Head out the door for that short walk or sit down on your ball. Chances are, once you've warmed up, you'll exercise for longer than you anticipated. Even if you don't, however, know that 10 minutes is better than nothing.

Exercise in the Morning   It's easy for the general stress and fatigue of a workday to make your brain believe that you don't have enough energy for your workout late in the day. Also, people are always competing for your time, and they may win out over your late-day exercise plans. Doing your ball workout first thing in the morning will make you feel good about your accomplishment for the rest of the day.

Change Your Location   You can do your ball workout anywhere, so move around. One day try it in front of the TV as you watch your favorite show. Another time do it in the backyard with the breeze on your face. Try it in different rooms in the house. Or head to the gym, where the other hard bodies will motivate you to work harder.

Set New Goals   Once you reach your initial goal, set new ones. If you've completely toned your tush, change your focus to a different body area. If you've mastered the basic exercises in chapter 2, move on to the more challenging ones in chapter 3.

I like to see how long I can balance on the ball in different positions. For example, I'll sit on the ball with my feet off the floor and watch the clock to see how long I last. Little self-contests like this keep me focused on constant improvement.

Buy a New Workout Outfit   If you wear it, you'll want to move in it. Whenever you think about skipping your workout, just put on your new workout clothes. Once you get dressed, you'll want to start moving.

Buy a Ball Video   You'll learn a whole new series of moves as well as gain additional ideas on how to best combine them. If possible, preview the video before buying, as some are extremely challenging. You want to find one at your level, not six levels above.

Take parts of what you learn from the video and incorporate them into your existing ball workouts—becoming the master of your own custom ball workout!

Listen to Music   Our favorite music has a way of making us want to move. On those days when you have trouble motivating yourself, put in a favorite CD and sit on your ball. You'll soon find yourself bouncing to the beat and doing your workout. The music may also help you throw in a few more reps.

Eat More Often   Many people feel too tired or too unmotivated to workout because of either too few or too many calories.

When you skip meals or don't eat often enough, your muscles and brain don't get enough fuel. When your brain runs low, it doesn't want you to move, and your motivation fades.

When you eat too much, you may feel like a nap rather than exercise. That's because your body diverts some of your blood volume away from your brain and muscles to your stomach to aid with digestion.

To avoid these problems, try to eat five small meals a day—a moderate breakfast, lunch, and dinner plus two small snacks at midmorning and midafternoon. Smaller, more frequent meals will give you a constant supply of energy and fuel your motivation all day long.

Drink a Glass of Water   When you are dehydrated, your brain suffers and your motivation plummets. Start your day with a glass or two of water, and follow up with a glass at every meal. Carry water bottles with you everywhere to remind yourself to drink.

Keep Your Ball in Plain View   If you see the exercise ball, you're more likely to get on it. A visual reminder is a powerful motivational force. Keep your ball in a place that you walk past often. Every time you see it, you'll be reminded of that workout you need to do today.

12

partner pointers

Your social network greatly influences whether
you'll stick with your new habits

Your social network of family and friends wields a lot of power, probably more than you realize. This support, or lack of it, can make all the difference in whether you stay with your fitness program for your lifetime.

Just consider this study of 3,342 adults from six different European countries. Those who felt their family, friends, coworkers, or boss supported their efforts were more than twice as likely to remain fit and active as those without this support. In another study, women were less likely to drop out of an exercise class if they felt support from the other members in the class.

Other surveys show that single mothers and other women with heavy care-giving responsibilities rank their family life as a primary reason for not exercising. On the other hand, women with husbands or extended families who share the child-rearing load are more apt to find the time to work out.

Other studies show that most women will stick with a new program if they perform it with a partner or with a group. They also tend to exercise more often and more consistently and feel more confident about their progress than those who exercise alone.

Married with Children?

Children can sometimes create a nonnegotiable obstacle to working out. There's simply no way a two-year-old understands when you say, "Mommy needs to workout so she'll stay fit and healthy for your entire life."

As every mother knows, when a toddler wants a piece of your time, he or she will find a way to get it. To fit in your workouts, particularly if you have small children, try these options.

- Do your ball workout at a fitness center. Most now offer daycare. As an added attraction, most centers provide full-length mirrors so you can check your form.

- Find a ball buddy who also has small children. As you do an exercise on the ball, she watches and entertains the toddlers. When she does her set, you watch the kids.

- Cordon off your child. Though the ball certainly provides a much safer form of strength training than dumbbells or barbells, you can still accidentally injure your child or yourself if you are not careful. You might be put off your balance by small objects in the path of the ball or your foot. You don't want to run the risk of rolling on top of your child. So use a playpen or other device that keeps your child a safe distance away from you and the ball—but still in sight.

- Try the rolling game. If your child wants attention—*now!*—try rolling the ball back and forth to your toddler between sets. Or, place the toddler on the ball, holding your child in place so he or she can't fall off. Toddlers find the exercise fun, and they improve their motor and balance skills as well.

This doesn't mean that you must get everyone you know—friends, husband, children—on the ball program (though that certainly wouldn't hurt!). It does mean that for optimal motivation, you must maximize your contact with people who support your efforts and minimize contact with those who do not.

Networking Skills

To create an exercise network, you first must come out of the fitness closet. Too often, when women start a new fitness and weight loss program, they don't tell anyone. They figure that if they fail, no one will know.

Although it may feel more comfortable to keep mum, this secrecy tends to work against you rather than for you and sets you up to fail.

Instead, I encourage you to tell everyone you know about your new habits and lifestyle. I don't know about you, but when I tell people I'm going to do something, I feel downright embarrassed if I don't follow through. Broadcasting the news gives me a strong sense of commitment to my fitness program.

The power of positive peer pressure can probably be seen most convincingly in Bill Bryson, the author of *A Walk in the Woods*. The noted travel writer and self-described couch potato decided one day that he would hike the Appalachian Trail, a 2,100-plus-mile hiking path that runs from Georgia to Maine. He told all his friends and colleagues about his plans *before* he researched the trip. To his dismay, he found that the hike would take months and that he would be hiking and camping in the wild, battling all sorts of dangers from bears to bugs to extreme weather. Faced with all these perils, he desperately wanted to change his mind. However, the fear of being seen as a quitter made him go ahead with his escapade, and he soon found himself in Georgia beginning the hike. Announcing his project ahead of time led him to complete it.

Let this same fear of becoming a quitter work to your advantage. That way when friends casually ask, "How's that ball program coming?" you can answer, "It's fantastic!"

Being open about your efforts will also help you more easily separate your supporters from your zappers. Yes, we all have people in our lives who not only fail to support our healthy habits but also sometimes work against our efforts. If you're overweight, you may encounter friends or family members who derive some personal self-esteem from you not succeeding. They may feel threatened by your weight loss and think that a skinnier you may not be as interested in spending time with a fatter them.

Others may selfishly focus on what they may lose from your new healthy habits. A mother, husband, or friend may feel jealous of the time you spend away from him or her with the exercise ball. Or, if you often went out for dessert or fries or other high-calorie, fattening foods with certain friends, they may miss the old "fun" you.

To overcome these saboteurs, make a list of the most important people in your life. This list should include anyone you live with, such as a roommate, husband, and children. It should also include anyone you spend a lot of time with, such as immediate family and close friends and co-workers.

Once you've listed everyone, think about what each person may gain or lose when you get fit and healthy. How did each respond when you revealed your new habits? Who was supportive and who wasn't?

Write an "S" next to people who have been supportive, who fuel your motivation, and compliment you on your efforts.

Write an "NS" next to those who are not supportive. Carefully look at these names and think about the reasons why they aren't supportive. Are they jealous? What do they have to lose by you becoming fit and healthy?

Once you've done this assessment, you must make a decision. Do you need to continue to spend time with everyone on your "NS" list? Exactly how close are you? Of course, some people on your NS list are nonnegotiable, notably your children and close family. But perhaps you could benefit from spending less time around the others. Remember, it's your health, it's your body. Stick up for your needs.

Next, confront the nonnegotiable people on your NS list. For example, if your husband isn't pulling his fair share of the household duties, you might explain to him how much better and sexier you feel when you exercise and that you need his help at creating time to fit in your workout.

As for those who feel jealous of the time you spend with the ball, reassure them that you still love them. Invite them over and have them work out with you.

As for your "food friends," think of pleasant ways you can spend time together without eating. Could you take a walk or go to a dance club together rather than talk over beer and nachos?

It may take a lot of work, but eventually you'll find that you can pull many from your "NS" list into your corner. Approaching these people in a positive way will help fuel your own motivation.

Expanding Your Network

After you've come to terms with family and friends, you may want to increase your chances of success even more by forging new networks with people who are already fit.

You might choose to work out with a partner, a ball buddy who will keep you honest. Studies show that women who do their exercises with partners are less likely to skip their workouts.

Before finding a workout buddy, however, carefully consider whether a partner will increase your chances of success. Although many people thrive on a social workout setting, others don't. If you like to fit in a workout during snippets of free time, don't like to talk as you work out, or feel embarrassed about your body size or shape, you may prefer to exercise alone.

However, if you enjoy being around others, tend to put off your workouts, and like working out at a set time, you will probably benefit from a buddy.

Here are some tips to help find the best workout partner.

Find Someone with Similar Goals   If you want to lose weight, choose a partner who also wants to slim down. If you want to become fit so that you can bolster your success at another sport, such as tennis or swimming, choose a partner who wants the same. That way you both can talk about your progress and more easily understand each other's needs and challenges.

Find Someone You Like   It doesn't matter if your partner is a man or a woman. You want someone you click with. If you don't like your partner's personality, you may start looking for excuses to cancel your workout dates.

Find Someone with Your Workout Philosophy   If you want to move through your workout efficiently within a half hour, you'll feel frustrated by a partner who spends half the time yakking and gossiping. On the other hand, if you don't mind if your workout takes an hour or more and you love social interaction, a chatty partner may be just what you need.

Find Someone Who Complements Your Motivation Level If you tend to procrastinate, you'll want a partner who likes to stick with the program. Your partner will keep you on task and not allow you to blow off your workout.

With these tips in hand, get out there, find your perfect workout buddy, and get started!

13

beautiful body, beautiful mind

Maximize your brainpower, and you'll also maximize
your motivation, happiness, and inner beauty

To maintain the benefits that you've reaped during the first six
weeks of your ball program, you must become fit from the inside
out. Once you change your inner world, you'll create an intrinsic
motivation that helps you meet your nutritional and fitness goals—
automatically.

Your first step involves learning to appreciate your inner and outer
beauty.

I'll be realistic. Starting an exercise program and eating more
healthfully will probably never make your body look like Cindy Craw-
ford's, Brittany Spears's, or Naomi Campbell's. However, that doesn't
mean you can't create a beautiful body.

Most of us women fall victim to the images we see on television,
the movie screen, and magazine covers. Research shows that the slender models and actresses we see over and over are abnormally thin.
One study of *Playboy* found that the centerfold models had body mass
indexes (a comparison of weight to height) of 18 or lower. Compare
this with a healthy woman's body mass index of 18.5 to 24.

Trying to achieve the look of these models will not only frustrate you but may also seriously harm your health. Research shows that being underweight is just as bad for your health as being overweight.

Also, don't think that these women come by their gorgeous figures naturally. Many augment their breasts with implants; skim fat off their tummies, butts, and thighs with regular liposuction treatments; and keep off the rest with super-low-calorie diets. Then, photographers and art directors manipulate the already rail-thin bodies to look even thinner by using computerized techniques that airbrush off any hint of cellulite or bulge.

Overcoming these media images isn't easy. One study found that young girls on the island of Fiji developed eating disorders and excessive interest in weight loss after seeing American television shows for the first time. A study in the United States found that excessive dieting and use of diet pills increase in direct correlation with the amount of time teenage girls spend reading beauty and fashion magazines.

To overcome poor body image, follow these tips.

Compare Yourself with Real People Start by comparing yourself with real women rather than the women you see on television or in the pages of magazines.

Focus on the Journey, Not the Destination Take your focus off the scale and the size of your thighs and put it on healthful eating and exercising. Congratulate yourself for daily accomplishments such as doing your ball workout consistently or eating more fruits and vegetables.

Stick with the Program Exercise is one of the best body image boosters around. Whenever you're feeling "fat," go for a walk. Getting your body moving boosts your mood and attitude toward yourself.

Compliment Your Body Rather than focusing on the areas of your body you don't like, focus on the ones you do like. Perhaps you have defined collarbones, small feet, or delicate fingers.

Beautiful Goals

Every year on January 2, people flood fitness centers, write out a check for a yearly membership, and resolve to start and stick with an exercise program.

For the first week, they show up nearly every day. The next week they do the same. As each week progresses, however, they come fewer and fewer times, until within a month or two, they fail to show up at all.

They fail because they set ugly goals.

Your goals can inspire you to stick with your program, or they can depress you so much that eventually you deflate the ball and go back to your life as a couch potato. One set of goals is realistic, the other is not. Here are some tips for realistic goal setting.

Take Baby Steps   If you've never exercised before, don't plan to do it three or more days a week. That's a goal that takes time and physical and mental commitment. Instead, try the ball workout just once a week. You might not even complete the entire workout. That's fine. Even if you just sit on the ball and read through the exercises, you've done more than you ever did before.

Focus on How You Feel, Not on the Scale   Don't try to create a body shape that is unrealistic. One woman recently complained to me of her frustration of not achieving a "cut" look. She weighed 115 pounds and worked out six days a week. Her workouts included 40 minutes of aerobics, 15 minutes of abdominal work, and another 50 minutes of weight training. She also ice-skated three times a week. She wanted to know what to add to her regimen to make her look "cut."

I told her the body fat that women store under their skin creates the smooth appearance that many of us associate with being female. Trying to achieve the muscle definition of a man is unrealistic for many women.

We are all born with a body type that stays with us all our lives. Trying to change it is not only frustrating but also impossible. I encourage you to focus your goals on your eating and exercise habits and other things you can control rather than on what you can't control, such as your body shape.

Develop the Art of Patience   Many women are strongly motivated at the beginning of a fitness program. During the first couple of weeks, healthful eating and exercising feel easy when fueled with such strong willpower. Maybe they try to achieve faster results by skipping meals, eating fewer servings than recommended, and exercising more often or longer than recommended.

Trying to overdo it in an attempt to get the pounds off yesterday will backfire. Skipping meals or eating fewer calories than recommended will soon slow your metabolism as your body cannibalizes muscle to make up for the shortfall. Then, when your willpower wanes and you return to eating normally, you'll gain weight. Also, when you overexercise, you run the risk of intense muscle soreness or even injury that could sideline you for a long period of time.

Weight loss takes time. Remember: Life is about joy. Fitness should be fun. Don't torture yourself. Enjoy and savor the journey to the new you.

Beautiful Thoughts

Take a moment to consider whether you are one of those people for whom a glass of water is "half empty" or "half full."

If you are a "half-empty," negative thinker, you'll experience a tougher time sticking with healthful eating and exercising. Research shows that self-confidence and positive thinking play a huge role in whether people stick with new healthy habits.

In an interesting study, researchers asked 103 preteen and teenage girls to cycle at the same speed for 20 minutes. The researchers tracked the participants' perceived exertion and other indicators of fatigue. Girls who had indicated more self-confidence before the exer-

Do It and Do It Early

Many of us procrastinate away our exercise time because we think negative thoughts about our energy levels, stress levels, and the overall daily grind. For example, let's say you planned to do your ball workout on Tuesday morning. When you awoke, you were worried about other tasks and told yourself, "I'll do the ball workout at lunch. I'm too busy right now." When lunch came, you told yourself, "I'm too busy right now; I'll do it after work." You see where this is going.

There are days when you will "too" yourself out of your workout, claiming to be too tired, too hungry, too busy, or too stressed. When those days come, remember to look at the big picture. That bad Tuesday was just one day out of a month of successful workouts. Fortunately, you can prevent yourself from "too-ing" yourself out of most of your workouts by sticking to a morning routine. Morning is the time when most people have their maximum energy and also have control over their schedule. Simply telling yourself when you wake up, "I can do this" will make the difference between getting out of bed or sleeping 15 extra minutes.

cise had lower exertion levels compared with the girls who were less confident about their abilities.

We all know that self-confidence and positive thinking aren't traits that we can build over night. You can guard against sabotaging yourself with negative thinking with the following tips.

Always Get Back on the Ball　Too many women toss their ball routines aside after missing just a couple sessions. They tell me, "I had a bad week and didn't exercise at all, so I just quit." Others who had been sticking to a healthful eating plan fall off the ball after one night of overindulgence. "I ate a huge hunk of cheesecake. Everything is ruined," they tell me.

Relax   Your body doesn't lose strength all that quickly. You can miss an entire week or two of ball workouts and still maintain most of your strength.

Also, overeating on just one occasion isn't going to ruin your healthy eating efforts. People gain weight by overeating every day for a year or more. Overeating by 500 calories will result in less than a quarter-pound of weight gain. That's hardly a reason to toss in the towel! Whenever you overeat or miss a few workouts, remind yourself that it's not as bad as it seems. You will recover—as long as you get back on the ball.

Leave the Past Behind   If you've started and stopped exercise programs before or if you failed at fitness during high school attempts, banish those thoughts. Leave the past in the past. Everyone can do the workout—including you. Forget about failed attempts at aerobic dance, skiing, or other pursuits. Focus on the *now* and on the budding fitness enthusiast inside you.

Go Through the Motions   My friend Karen came to me many times after I taught her the ball workout and said to me, "I just don't think I'm doing it right." Yet, when I watched her do the workout, she did the exercises flawlessly.

If you've never exercised before, the ball workout will feel awkward. That doesn't mean you're doing it wrong. Rather it means your muscles are learning a new way of moving. Over time, the movement will feel more natural.

In the meantime, take steps to fuel your confidence. First, learn to trust your body. Focus on your muscles as you do your workout. Can you feel the muscles working? If you can, you're doing the exercise correctly. You can also invite a friend over to puzzle out the exercise together. If you both feel it should look a certain way, you're probably right. Finally, take comfort in knowing that there's no wrong way to exercise on the ball. If you do an exercise slightly differently from the way I recommend in this book, you merely run the risk of working a different muscle than you intended. You're still getting a workout!

Beautiful Eating

When you think of "emotional eating," you might imagine a 300-pound guest on an afternoon talk show wiping away tears as she explains how she eats to numb the pain from a past trauma. However, you don't need to have a tragic background like childhood abuse or any other traumatic event to eat emotionally. We *all* do it.

When was the last time you got really mad at your boss? Did you turn to food? When your son came home with straight A's, did you celebrate with pizza? Food has a way of calming our emotions, helping us celebrate a success or drown a sorrow, or just procrastinate over an assignment at work.

Comfort foods like chocolate and mashed potatoes contain ingredients that influence our brain chemistry almost like antidepressant and anti-anxiety medications.

Conversely, your mood can influence your appetite and desire to eat. In response to stressful situations, tiny glands near the kidneys produce a hormone called cortisol that may stimulate eating.

Here are some of the most common types of food we turn to in times of stress, depression, sadness, and even celebration, as well as what the research says about how they may alter chemicals in the brain.

Carbohydrates   Eating carbohydrate-rich foods, such as mashed potatoes, boosts insulin levels that, in turn, facilitate the entry into the brain of an amino acid called tryptophan. Tryptophan converts into a brain chemical called serotonin. Increased levels of serotonin may ease feelings of stress or anxiety.

Sugar   Although sugar is a type of carbohydrate, it affects mood through a different mechanism. Studies done on animals suggest that eating sugar can lower levels of the stress hormone cortisol. In one study, laboratory rats that were forced to swim in cold water and given sugar water to drink had lower levels of cortisol than did rats offered plain water.

Chocolate   Chocolate's small amounts of caffeine and another stimulant called theobromine wake up the brain and may mildly improve mood. Another compound in chocolate called phenylethylamine (PEA) lifts depression.

Food certainly works at soothing us and altering our moods. But when we use food as a brain drug too often, we notice the effects on our thighs, butts, and waistlines.

To overcome triggers that set off emotional eating, find a substitute for eating. Keep a food/mood journal. In it keep track of what you eat, when you eat it, your feelings of hunger (did you eat out of true hunger or emotional hunger), how you felt, whom you were with, and the circumstances of the past few hours.

Keep in mind that not all emotional eating centers on a negative emotion. You may eat more at dinner because the food symbolizes the love you feel for your spouse. Or, you may eat more when out with friends because the food compliments your already buoyed feelings.

Your food/mood journal will help you develop the habit of pausing and thinking before you eat. Take it one step further. After one week, look over your entries. Try to puzzle out the patterns to your eating. On a separate piece of paper, write down the top four or five situations where you find you ate foods you wish you hadn't.

Next to each situation, write down how you can circumvent this kind of eating. If you tend to overeat when you go out with your friends, you might plan an activity not centered on food. How about a night of dancing or miniature golf?

If you tend to reward yourself with food after a long day at the office, choose a massage or bubble bath instead.

Another good alternate activity: exercising. Studies show that a single session of exercise can dramatically lift one's mood. Calling a friend may also help. Often simply talking about your bad day can help you calm down before you turn to food.

Once you've come up with alternatives to eating, follow this process whenever you catch yourself eating when you're not really hungry.

1. Ask yourself, "How do I feel?" Awareness of your emotional triggers is half the battle.

2. Write it down. Jot down your thoughts—what you wanted to say to your boss but didn't—or anything else that may help you settle your nerves.

3. Look over your replacement list and find a replacement activity that will help you feel better without the help of food.

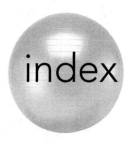

index

A

Abdominals
    back problems and, 19–20
    Ball Crunches, 47
    Classic Crunches, 31–32
    core vs., 25–26
    gaining fat in, 95–96
    Oblique Twist, 78–79
    Side-Ups, 59
    spot work for, 22, 258
Adenosine triphosphate (ATP), 133–134
Aerobics, 129–135. *See also* Walking
    workouts
    for calorie and fat burning, 98, 130
    during rest breaks, 197
    feeling better during, 133–134
    jogging, 131–132
    metabolism and, 129
    warm up and cool down, 134–135
Age, xiii, xiv, xv
Alternating Flies, 80–81
Appetite, 130, 277
Arms, 65, 258
Around the World Stretch, 15, 260
Atlas Lunge, 68

B

Back (lower)
    Standing Torso Twist, 60
    Torso Life and Twist, 82
    Upper Torso Lift, 33–34
    X Marks the Spot, 48, 260
Back problems, 19–20, 25, 54, 247
Back (upper)
    Alternating Flies, 80–81
    Kneeling Back Flies, 35
    Off-The-Ball Back Flies, 61–62
    Stomach Back Flies, 49–50, 265
Ball Crunches, 47
Balldynamics.com, 4, 24, 25
Ball Fighting, 261
Balls. *See* Fitness balls
Ball Tapping, 262
Barbells, 20
Basic body positions, 8–13
    Bridge, 10
    Incline Bridge, 9
    neutral spine for, 7, 248
    Prone Bridge, 12
    Prone Drape, 11
    Reverse Bridge, 13

Basic Program, 27–70. *See also* Basic body
    positions; Warm-up stretches
  overview, xvi–xix, 27–30
  warm-up stretches, 14–18, 260
  Week 1 and 2, 31–46
  Week 3 and 4, 47–58
  Week 5 and 6, 59–70
Biceps
  Bridge-Back Curls, 51
  Off-The-Ball Curls, 63, 83
  Preacher Ball Curls, 36–37
Big and Little Squeezes, 259
Body image, 93, 95, 205, 297–298,
    299–300
Boredom, 29, 72, 73, 132–133, 287
Breakfast, 278, 283
Breast exercises, 64
Breath, synchronizing, 29
Bridge, 10
Bridge-Back Curls, 51
Bridge Triceps Press, 58
Bryson, Bill, 293
Buddha Stretch, 17, 260
Burst-resistance, 20–21
Butt Lift, 44, 76
Butt Lift and Curl, 272
Buttocks. *See* Legs (butt/calves)

C
Caffeine, 116
Calf Raises, 55
Calories
  aerobic exercise and, 129
  burning, xv, 188, 195, 197
  calorie counters, 104
  cutting, 99, 173, 175, 200, 219
  eyeballing portions, 104, 106, 117, 121
  sample eating charts/menus for, 121–127
  for specific desserts, 109–110
  weight loss and, 102, 103–104, 106–107
Calves. *See* Legs (butt/calves)
Carbohydrates, 114–115, 118, 303
Cardiovascular exercise. *See* Aerobics

Challenging exercises
  abdominals, 78–79
  back, 80–82
  biceps, 83
  chest, 84
  as confidence builders, 72–73
  core exercises, 85
  legs, 86–87, 88
  motivation and, 192
  shoulders, 89
  tips for creating, 73–76, 135, 158
  triceps, 90
Cheating, 180
Chest
  Chest Flies, 52
  Chest-Press Incline, 64
  One-Legged Chest Fly Incline, 84
  Push-Ups, 38–39, 265
Children. *See also* Family and friends
  fitness balls for, ix, 6
  Kneeling Layouts with, 53
  rolling game with, 292
  safety issues for, 21, 292
  workouts with, 260–262
Chip Shot, 264
Chocolate, 281, 304
Classic Crunches, 31–32
Clothing, 144, 154, 183, 231, 239, 288
Commitment, 138, 293
Confidence, 71–72, 300–301, 302–303.
    See also Challenging exercises
Core body strength
  Arm-Swing Rolls, 65
  described, 25–26
  fitness balls and, xii, 253
  Jackknifes, 85
  Knee Fold-Ups, 40–41
  Kneeling Layouts, 53
Customized routines
  creating your own, 245–252
  for family and friends, 260–262
  fifteen minute workouts, 254–257
  for golfers, 263–264
  Muscle Memory chart for, 74

for runners, 271–272
for snow sports, 267–268
for swimmers, 265–266
for tennis players, 269–270
trouble spot workouts, 257–259

D

Dessert, 101–110
calories, 107, 118
choosing, 107–109
Dessert Diet food pyramids, 106–107, 119–121
list of common types, 109–110
weight-loss and, 101–102
Diet. *See also* Calories; Dessert; Servings
carbohydrates, 114–115, 118, 303
charts/menus, 121–127
discovering new foods, 168, 185
emotional eating, 303–305
fats, 113–114, 118, 175
fish, 118, 209
fluids, 115–116, 277
Food Diary, 105
improving, 236
maintaining, 286
meat, 118, 219
overeating, 130, 173, 226, 275, 289, 302
protein, xvi, 111–112
shopping tip, 202
snacks, 226
stress and, 280–282
traveling and, 278–279
weight loss and, 98–99
Dietwatch.com, 104
Double Push-Offs, 266
Drop Squat Shoulder Press, 255–257
Dumbbells, xi, xii, xiii, 4, 20, 24

E

Eating charts/menus, 121–127
Eating out, 173, 276–277
Emotions, 182, 230, 296, 303–305

Errand walks, 166
External Rotation on Ball, 270

F

Family and friends, 217, 260–262, 294. *See also* Children
Fat
abdominal fat, 95–96
burning, 98, 130, 132
female fat cells, 94–96, 98
omega-3 fatty acids, 113
recipes, removing fat from, 175
saturated fat, 113
servings of, 118
Fat-free foods, 99
Fatigue, "good," 14
Fat storage, 95–96, 131
Fifteen minute workouts, 254–259
Fish, 118, 209
Fitness balls. *See also* Heavy balls
awkwardness with, 141
basic body positions for, 7–13
benefits of, 3, 97
burst-resistance of, 20–21
kneeling on, 7, 252
pumping up, 24–25
purchasing, 5, 24, 25
sitting on, 6–7, 178, 251–252
sizes of, 4–5
traveling with, xii–xiii, 280
types of, 4–5
Fluids, 115–116, 277
Flying Carpet, 69
Food Diary, 105
Friends and family, 217, 260–262, 294. *See also* Children
Frozen dinners, 279
Fruits, 118, 278–279

G

Goal setting, 288, 299–300
Golf, 14, 263–264
Gymnic balls, 4–5, 20

H

Hamstring Curls, 42–43, 76
Health issues, for starting workout, 7–8
Heart disease, 96
Heavy balls, 4–5, 19, 24
Hormone sensitive lipase (HSL), 95
Hyperextension, 248

I

Incline Bridge, 9
Inner coach, 247, 249

J

Jackknifes, 85
Jogging, 131–132

K

Knee Fold-Ups, 40–41
Kneeling Back Flies, 35
Kneeling Layouts, 53
Kneeling on fitness balls, 7
Knee pain, 54

L

Lateral Lifts, 89
Lean muscle look, xiii, 14, 23, 246
Legs (butt/calves)
    Atlas Lunge, 68
    Butt Lift, 44, 76
    Butt Lift and Curl, 272
    Calf Raises, 55
    One-Leg Drop Squat, 88
Legs (thighs)
    Big and Little Squeezes, 259
    Drop Squats, 54
    Hamstring Curls, 42–43, 76
    Scissors Lift, 86–87
    Seated Leg Stretch, 18
    spot work for, 257–259
    Thigh Buster, 66–67

Lifting and twisting, 248
Lipoprotein lipase (LPL), 94
Listening to your body, 8, 14, 20
Low Body Stretch, 16, 260
Lunch, 283–284

M

Massage, 224
Mats, 5
Meal planning, 190
Meat, 118, 219
Medicine balls, 24
Menopause, 95–96
Menu samples, 123–127
Metabolism
    aerobics and, 129
    age and, xiv, xv
    diet and, 99
    strength training and, xiv–xv
    total body workout and, 23, 97, 246–247
    undereating and, 300
Motivation. *See also* Boredom; Challenging
        exercises
    challenges and, 192
    clothing and, 144, 154, 183, 231, 239, 288
    exercise partners for, 291, 292, 293
    maintaining, 285–289
    overcoming resistance and, 154
    tips for, 99–100, 146
    waning of, 179
"Muscle failure," 75
Muscle Memory chart, 74
Muscles
    adding reps and weight, 75
    alternating workouts for, 23
    calories burned by, xiv, xv
    changing body positions and, 75–76
    "good" fatigue and, 14
    major muscle groups, 246
    pre-exhausting, 73
    soreness, 22
    total body workout vs. spot work, 23, 97,
        246–247

working opposing muscle groups, 75, 250
workout chart for, 74
Music, 229, 288

N

Negative thinking, 133
Networking, 293–296
Neutral spine, 7, 248

O

Obliques, 26
Oblique Twist, 78–79
Off-The-Ball Back Flies, 61–62
Off-The-Ball Curls, 63, 83
Omega-3 fatty acids, 113
One-Leg Drop Squat, 88
One-Legged Chest Fly Incline, 84
One-Legged Triceps Ball Press, 90
Opposing muscles, 75
Overeating, 130, 173, 226, 275, 289, 302
Overexercising, 300

P

Pain. *See also* Safety issues
    during aerobics, 131–132
    during workouts, 7–8, 248
    knee pain, 54
    shoulder blade pain, 35
Partners for working out, 291–296
Patience, 300
Pedometers, 166
Pets, 21–22
Pilates, 250
Portions. *See* Servings
Positions. *See* Basic body positions
Positive thinking, 161, 300–301
Posture, xii, 7, 248
Power center. *See* Core body strength
Preacher Ball Curls, 36–37
Problem-solving walks, 171
Procrastination, 301

Prone Bridge, 11
Prone Drape, 10
Protein, xvi, 111–112
Pumps, 24–25
Push-Offs, 45, 260, 266
Push-Ups, 38–39, 265

R

Recipes, removing fat from, 175
Rectus abdominus, 26, 31, 47
Relaxation, 156, 173
Restaurants, 173, 276–277
Rest breaks
    aerobics during, 197, 249–250
    eliminating, 250, 254, 255
    importance of, 22–23, 29–30, 207
Reverse Bridge, 13
Right-Angle Lateral Lifts, 56–57
Rubber tubing, 280
Running, 18, 132, 271–272

S

Saboteurs, 294–295
Safety issues
    for barbells, 20
    burst-resistance of fitness balls, 20–21
    for children, 21, 292
    dropping heavy balls, 8
    falling off the ball, 20
    pets and, 21–22
    tips for, 7–8, 248
Salad bars, 279
Salt, 282
Saturated fat, 113
Scheduling/planning workouts, 171, 222,
    241, 280, 301
Scissors Lift, 86–87
Seated Leg Stretch, 18
Serotonin, 102, 303
Servings
    eating half portions, 173, 276
    eyeballing, 104, 106, 117, 121
    for specific foods, 118

Sex hormones, 95
Shoes, 149, 279
Shoulders
    building up, 97
    Double Push-Offs, 266
    Flying Carpet, 69
    Lateral Lifts, 89
    pain in, 35
    Push-Offs, 45, 260
    Right-Angle Lateral Lifts, 56–57
Side-Ups, 59
Silence, 151
Six-Week Workout, 137–241. *See also* Basic
        Program; Walking workouts
    preparing for, 137–139
    strength-training and, 97–98
    Week 1, 140–156
    Week 2, 157–173
    Week 3, 174–190
    Week 4, 191–207
    Week 5, 208–224
    Week 6, 225–241
Skiing, 267–268
Snacks, 226
Snowboarding, 267–268
Snow sports, 267–268
Socializing
    exercise partners and, 291, 292, 293,
        295–296
    networking, 293–296
    walking and, 163
Soft drinks, 116
Space for workouts, 7, 8, 248
Speed, 75–76, 131–132
Spine, neutral position, 7, 248
Spot reducing. *See* Trouble spots
Spotting, 24
Sprinting, 132
Squats
    Drop Squats, 54
    Drop Squat Shoulder Press,
        255–257
    knee pain and, 54

    One-Leg Drop Squat, 88
    Wall Squats, 268
Standing Torso Twist, 60
Starvation mode, 103, 300
Steroids, xvi
Stomach Back Flies, 49–50, 265
Stopwatch, 188
Strength training, xiv–xvi, 97–98, 207
Stress, 280–282
Stretches. *See* Warm-up stretches
Sugar, 304
Swimming, x, xi, 265–266

T

Telephones, cordless, 212
Tennis, 269–270
Thighs. *See also* Legs (thighs)
    losing fat from, 95
Thoughts, positive, 161, 300–301
Torso Life and Twist, 82
Transverse abdominus, 26
Travel, xii–xiii, 25, 278–279, 280
Triceps
    Bridge Triceps Press, 58
    One-Legged Triceps Ball Press, 90
    Triceps Ball Press, 46
    Triceps Extension, 70, 265
Trouble spots
    abdominal spot work, 22, 258
    customized routines for, 257–259
    legs (thighs) work, 257–259
    targeting, 23, 251
    total body workout and, 23, 97,
        246–247
    upper arm work, 258
Tryptophan, 303
Twisting exercises
    cautions for, 248
    Chip Shot, 264
    Oblique Twist, 78–79
    Standing Torso Twist, 60
    Torso Life and Twist, 82

U

Undereating, 103, 300
Underweight, 298
Upper arms, 258
Upper Torso Lift, 33–34

V

Variety, importance of, 29, 73, 97–98, 249
Vegetables, 118
Videos, 288

W

Walking workouts
    10-minutes, 144, 149, 154
    15-minutes, 161, 166, 171
    20-minutes, 178, 183, 188, 195
    25-minutes, 205
    30-minutes, 212, 217, 222
    35-minutes, 200, 229, 234, 239
    counting steps during, 166
    getting the most from, 136–137
    as social time, 163
    weight-loss with, 98, 134
A Walk in the Woods, 293
Wall Squats, 268
Warm up and cool down, 134–135
Warm-up stretches
    Around the World, 15, 260
    Buddha Stretch, 17, 260
    children and, 260
    Low Body Stretch, 16, 260
    Seated Leg Stretch, 18

Water, 277, 289
Weight benches, 20
Weight loss
    aerobic exercise for, 129
    calories and, 102, 103–104, 106–107
    cautions for, 207
    dessert and, 101–102
    gauging progress in, 234
    maintaining, 130
    repeated lose and gain, 131
    underweight, 298
    walking and, 98, 134
Weight machines, xii, xiii
Weights, 14, 214
Work, eating at, 282–284
Workouts. See also Basic Program;
        Customized routines; Six-Week
        Workout
    benefits of, 153
    expectations for, xviii–xix
    increasing effectiveness of, 214
    main body areas targeted, 28
    missing, 23, 301–302
    scheduling/planning, 171, 222, 241,
        280, 301
    time needed for, 252, 253

X

X Marks the Spot, 48, 260

Y

Yoga, 250

about the author

Liz Applegate, Ph.D., nationally renowned expert on nutrition and fitness, is a faculty member at the University of California, Davis. Her enthusiasm and informal teaching style make her undergraduate nutrition classes the nation's largest, with enrollment exceeding 2,000 annually. She is a recent recipient of the Excellence in Teaching Award from the University of California.

Dr. Applegate is also a columnist and nutrition editor for *Runner's World* magazine and is on the editorial board of the *International Journal of Sports Nutrition.* She is the author of several books on fitness and nutrition and has written more than 300 articles for national magazines such as *Woman's Day, Better Homes and Gardens, Good Housekeeping,* and others.

A Fellow of the American College of Sports Medicine, Dr. Applegate is also a member of the Sports, Cardiovascular, and Wellness Nutritionists, a practice group of the American Dietetic Association, and on the board of directors of the American Council on Exercise (ACE). Frequently serving as a keynote speaker at industry, athletic, and scientific meetings, she has been a guest on more than 200 international, national, and local radio and television shows, including *Good Morning America* and health segments on CNN and ESPN. Dr. Applegate serves as a nutrition consultant for the U.S. Olympic Team as well as NBA and NFL individuals and teams. She lives in Davis, California.

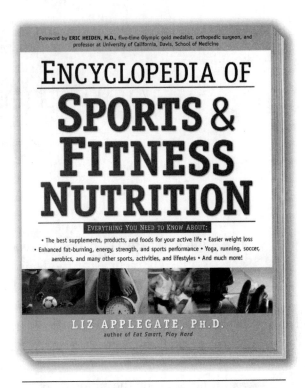